THESE CAN MAKE YOU ILL

NOT ALL IN THE MIND

Dr. Richard Mackarness

Publishing by BN Publishing

www.bnpublishing.com

info@bnpublishing.com

For information regarding special discounts for bulk purchases, please contact BN Publishing at

sales@bnpublishing.net

To my friend and colleague
Dr Ted Randolph of Chicago, who taught me
most of what I know of this subject,
in affection and respect

Surely the time has come to put away the notion that psychiatry deals just with mind disease . . . only in Wonderland can we find the grin without the cat.

FOSTER KENNEDY
Professor of Neurology, Cornell University 1936

Acknowledgements

As this book has taken me seventeen years to write, it is impossible to thank all the people who have helped me and whose work has influenced my thinking and practice, so I hope that any omissions in this acknowledgement will be forgiven.

The book is dedicated to Dr Ted Randolph of Chicago who has been friend, teacher and colleague to me ever since I was first introduced to him by his brother-in-law Dr Donald Mitchell in 1958. Many other doctors, here and in America, have helped me since with advice and guidance and I would single out for particular mention Dr Marshall Mandell of New York who taught me how to use the sublingual provocative food test, the late Dr Herbert Rinkel of Kansas City who explained the phenomenon of masking in food allergy to me, and the late Dr Albert Rowe of Oakland, San Francisco, who showed me over his food allergy clinic in 1963 and told me about his elimination diets. These men gave me the background on which to work.

Coming to more recent times, I wish to thank Professor Truelove of Oxford for confirming verbally to me his findings on the role of milk in provoking attacks of ulcerative colitis and for permission to quote from his published work on the subject in the *British Medical Journal*. Grateful thanks also to the editor of that journal for permission to quote. Particular thanks to Dr John Lyon, Consultant Psychiatrist at my own hospital, for the encouragement and facilities he has given me to carry out research here at Park Prewett, and to the staff of the Psychiatric Intensive Care Unit which John Lyon founded. The healthy scepticism of my other medical and psychiatric colleagues must be acknowledged also, for it has been one of the biggest spurs to my endeavours and has helped to keep my feet on the ground. Now that some of them are referring patients to me for the treatment described in this book I must acknowledge my debt to those nurses who have helped me most to carry the treatments through: Sister Williams on the Mother-and-Baby Unit, and Sister Chu and Staff Nurse Todd on Chute Ward. Several general practitioners in the North Hampshire Area have given me valuable support, not only by referring patients but by understanding my methods and seeing that the patients followed them after discharge from hospital.

I am grateful for the backing and encouragement given to me by Professor Martin, Chairman of the Wessex Clinical Research Committee, and to the various committees in Basingstoke which have supported my research work and have seen to it that I now have my own out-patient clinic at the Basingstoke District Hospital in which to study and treat patients suffering from the effects of allergy to commonly encountered foods and chemicals. Dr John Fowler, Consultant Physician at Basingstoke, has been especially helpful, as have the two Out-Patient Sisters: Sister Jones and Sister Price. Mrs Yorke, the Allergy Sister, has been most helpful in doing skin tests for me and the Chief Pharmacist, Mr Fennell, has gone to endless trouble to put up allergen-free versions of drugs I have wished to prescribe. Mr Wadley, the Catering Officer, and the Dieticians who work with him have done more on a day-to-day basis than anyone else to make my work possible. And before coming to the end of these personal acknowledgements I must mention the patients themselves, particularly 'Joanna', many of whom have put themselves and their relatives to much trouble and personal expense in order to follow my instructions and keep themselves well. To see and hear from them has been a continual encouragement and a valuable check on the methods I have been using. Some of the patients I treated in general practice between 1958 and 1965, when I went into psychiatry, still keep in touch with me and it is a pleasure to hear of the progress they have been making.

Formal acknowledgements are made to the following authors and their publishers for direct quotations which I have used:

Dr John Fry: *Common Diseases – Their Nature, Incidence and Care*, Medical and Technical Publications Ltd (Lancaster); Professor Hans Selye and *Nature*; Dr Francis Adams: *The Genuine Works of Hippocrates*, Williams and Wilkins Company, Baltimore;
the late Dr Blake Donaldson: *Strong Medicine*, Doubleday (New York) and Cassell (London);
Dr F. Curtis Dohan and the *British Journal of Psychiatry*;
Dr George L. Thorpe and the *Journal of the American Medical Association*;
Dr T. G. Randolph: *Human Ecology and Susceptibility to the Chemical Environment*, Charles C. Thomas, Springfield, Illinois.

Finally, my secretary Marjory Hurst who has been an unfailing support to me, and my wife and son who have put up with my working on this book for so many years without getting bored with the subject.

R.M.
Basingstoke District Hospital
(Psychiatric Division)
1975

Publisher's note

Explanatory footnotes appear at the bottom of the page; references indicated by numbers in the text can be found at the back of the book on pages 149–51.

Introduction

'Modern medicine has become a major threat to health and its potential for social, even physical, disruption is rivalled only by the perils inherent in the industrialized production of food.'

When Ivan Illich said this in 1974, he was putting into words two of the worst and so far largely unspoken fears of doctors in developed countries today.

Not only are British and American doctors unable to make a clear diagnosis in up to one half of the patients who come to consult them, but because of this, most of the treatments they have to offer are for the control of symptoms only, not for the eradication of the causes of disease, which still elude them. In spite of the increasingly sophisticated methods of investigation available to hospital specialists and general practitioners, the practice of medicine often remains at best ineffective from the patient's point of view, and at worst positively harmful: huge volumes are now published on iatrogenic disease – disease arising as an unwanted by-product of modern medical treatment, particularly with drugs.

Dr John Fry, a famous GP practising at Beckenham, near London, who was one of the prime movers in the foundation of the Royal College of General Practice, describes in his book *Common Diseases – Their Nature, Incidence and Care*[15] the three shocks awaiting the newly hospital-qualified doctor entering general practice. Shock number one is 'The rude awakening that comes to the physician on entering the field of primary care and practice . . . to be faced with a mass of apparently unrecognized, undefinable and unfamiliar emotional disorders.' Shock number two comes with the realization that cure is almost impossible in these conditions, and number three – a terrible thing for the scientifically and academically trained modern physician – with the realization that emotional disorders cannot be categorized neatly like blood disorders, nor labelled or diagnosed with any accuracy at all.

By 'emotional disorders' Dr Fry means those disorders which manifest themselves as disturbances of thought, feeling and behaviour. These are properly the province of the psychiatrist but as there are not nearly enough psychiatrists to go round, the GP usually has to try to deal with them himself – an impossible task when he has no idea how they arise. And when you add to what Fry calls emotional illnesses the host of other equally mysterious diseases that affect the body rather than the behaviour, it is small wonder that doctors have the highest suicide rate of any profession or trade. Allergies, migraine, high blood pressure, heart attacks, bowel disorders and people who come saying they 'feel sick all over' mystify the modern doctor every day, and although the drug companies give him every kind of chemical to prescribe for the mitigation of symptoms, he must realize in his heart of hearts that he is still pouring drugs of which he knows little into patients of whom he knows even less – a cynical but profoundly true remark made about doctors many years ago, long before the era of 'scientific' medicine.

So we come to the second half of Ivan Illich's quote: the perils inherent in the industrialized production of food. Could this be one of the keys to the doctors' dilemma? That the food we eat is now so refined, processed and adulterated with chemicals that it is causing all or most of these new and strange epidemics, through our failure to adapt to it and stay healthy? I think this is more than a possibility. I think it is one important answer, and in this book I have tried to set out the evidence, based on my own clinical experience as a doctor and psychiatrist and on the experience and research of the growing band of medical men all over the world, who agree with this point of view and are trying to do something constructive about it before it is too late.

Although there has been no important advance in psychiatry since the introduction of the anti-depressant drugs in the 1950s, nothing in this book is intended to discredit the present methods used by doctors and psychiatrists. Instead, it offers them a new way of looking at the mysterious change that has overtaken the pattern of mental and physical illness now afflicting Western man.

part one

chapter one

At eleven o'clock on Wednesday morning 23 May 1973 Joanna sat in the doctors' lounge of Park Prewett Hospital, her eyes fixed on the floor, too anxious and depressed to say a word. She was being 'presented' at the weekly clinical case conference of the hospital, which is the psychiatric division of the Basingstoke and District General Hospital in England.

The routine at these weekly case conferences is always the same. The three clinical teams present a case in turn, choosing one which is unusually difficult from either the diagnostic or the management standpoint. After introductory remarks by the consultant in charge, the registrar or the assistant psychiatrist gives the case history, backed up by reports from the social worker, occupational therapist and clinical psychologist. The audience asks questions, then the patient is brought in and presented – quite an ordeal for the patient as a rule, although the manic, hysterical or psychopathic ones seem to enjoy it.

Joanna's case history had been presented to the audience of psychiatrists, medical students and psychiatric social workers by Dr John Lyon, consultant psychiatrist, Dr Ali Khan, his registrar, and the author, one of the six assistant psychiatrists at the hospital. However, she was so tense and unhappy that Dr Lyon let her go back to the ward after less than two minutes.

Joanna's first attack had come in October 1967, after the birth of her third child, when she had become irritable, tense, depressed, unable to feed the baby and occasionally violent towards the two older children. She had been treated for this attack by ECT at the Mayday Hospital in Croydon before she moved to North Hampshire early in 1968. At that time, she weighed about eleven stone but now, in May 1973, she was over fourteen stone. In the interval, she had been admitted to Park Prewett Hospital thirteen times, often compulsorily because the various psychiatrists called by the general practitioner to see her at home had considered her a danger to her children and herself. In her most disturbed phases she would slash her forearms with any nearby sharp object, not with definite suicidal intent, but as a way of relieving, if only temporarily, the unbearable tension and irritability mounting inside her. These wounds usually needed stitching and left deep scars, quite unlike the superficial scratches made by hysterical people indulging in attention-seeking suicidal gestures.

On one occasion, Joanna had knocked her three-and-a-half-year-old son unconscious, and on another had thrown her elder daughter through a closed window – luckily on the ground floor. Surprisingly, her three children had never shown any resentment towards their mother for their ill-treatment, seeming to realize with the clear, non-verbal insight of childhood that she could not help herself and loved them in spite of her repeated violence and neglect. Her husband showed the patience of a saint and stuck to her through seven terrible years.

Most of the psychiatrists at Park Prewett have had Joanna under their care at one time or another. Almost every diagnostic label in the book has been attached to her illness: schizophrenia, schizo-affective psychosis, presenile dementia, temporal lobe epilepsy, neurotic depression and anxiety hysteria.

In 1969, our clinical psychologist supported the two last-named diagnoses with this report, summarized in his delightful psychological jargon:

Psychopathology – failure of identification with beating behaviour, Performance IQ 86. Verbal IQ 96. Full scale IQ 91 (dull normal)
Projective tests: could not see much ... loneliness themes ... wanting to escape.
Rorschach: dull, unimaginative, avoids the situation, somatizes anxiety.
Diagnosis: neurotic depression with anxiety/hysteria.

The hospital psychiatric social worker who visited Joanna at home reported that the baby was scarcely ever taken out of its pram and its nappy was seldom changed. The children's department of the Local Authority had also been involved with Joanna and her children for a long time and spent many hours in conference with the psychiatrists in an attempt to solve her problems. Time after time it was almost decided to take the children into care, but the extraordinary resilience and contentedness of the boy and two little girls made it seem better to leave them at home, and some compromise was always devised to avoid this final step.

In his painstaking biography of Joanna, Dr Khan the Registrar brought out some unusual things. Her father, a railway man all his life, had died of cancer of the brain eight years earlier, at the age of sixty-one. Her mother had died two years later of cancer of the liver. Whereas her father had been kind, quiet and sympathetic, her mother had been distinctly unfriendly. Very strict, she had frequently hit Joanna, whose response was invariably to cry

19

and retire to her room. However, in spite of this ill-treatment, she shared her mother's bed to the age of eighteen, when she met and married her husband. Asked if she resented her mother, Joanna replied flatly: 'No. I still loved her.'

Joanna's own sex life was happy until the birth of her third child in the sixth year of her marriage. Then she progressively lost interest in sex so that during the last year there had been no intercourse with her husband or with anyone else. Stoically, her husband accepted this as part of the illness. Three years ago, at Park Prewett, Joanna struck up a relationship with a somewhat inadequate male patient. There was no physical sex and her husband did not try to interfere. Although strongly tempted, Joanna eventually decided not to leave her family for this man: 'because of the children and Donald [her husband] . . . because he has been so nice to me.' When she was asked her ambitions in life by Dr Khan, who was taking her biography, she replied, 'To have good health. To go home. To be happy.' Very normal ambitions after seven years of disabling psychotic illness. On her plans for the future, when asked just before the May '73 conference, she said, 'I wish to go home and be with my husband and children. But I can't see any hope of it.'

After Joanna had left the room with the nurse, Dr Lyon asked the meeting for their opinions and suggestions.

Almost without exception, leucotomy was recommended. All the doctors were gloomy about the outlook. The three children would be taken permanently into care. They were prompted mainly in their opinions by the fact that two or three weeks of concentrated effort by the staff of the Psychiatric Intensive Care Unit had failed to effect any improvement at all, and by her long history of thirteen admissions with failure to respond more than

20

briefly to every known combination of psychotropic drugs as well as several courses of ECT.

In this desperate situation I felt nothing could be lost by suggesting that Joanna might be a particularly severe case of food allergy and asking to be allowed to try and rehabilitate her. Everyone agreed it could do no harm and that everything even remotely possible should be tried before sending her to the neurosurgeons, though one or two were sceptical. So Dr Lyon told me Joanna could stay in the Intensive Care Unit and that he and his staff would give me every facility.

The idea that allergy or intolerance to certain foods can cause illness is not new. It was mentioned in the writings of Hippocrates and was revived by several American doctors, including Dr Albert Rowe, a physician in California in the 1920s and '30s. Rowe designed what he called elimination diets, which left out all foods of one particular kind, such as cereal grains or citrus fruits. Feeding these diets in rotation to patients, he was able to connect the disappearance of such chronic symptoms as headache, depression, nasal catarrh, irritable colon and day-long fatigue with the elimination of a food or group of foods. Arthur Coca of New Jersey and Herbert Rinkel of Kansas City were among those who confirmed and extended Rowe's work, while Ted Randolph in Chicago extended his research to include the chemical contaminants of food, air and water. Randolph also introduced the five-day fast at the beginning of an investigation, persuading the patient to fast for five days in a fume-free atmosphere on nothing but spring water (bottled if necessary). This method can be used on patients at home or in the hospital (I have tried both), in bed or out. If the symptoms do not diminish during the fast, then the illness is not due to food allergy.

If they do diminish, the next step is individual food ingestion tests, in which the patient is given test feedings of single foods he has eaten often in the past, and is then watched for an acute return of the symptoms. These usually recur within an hour or two and sometimes within minutes. The individual food ingestion test was developed by Rinkel, who found Rowe's rotating elimination tests too cumbersome.

I first encountered the field of food allergy in 1958, when I stayed with Dr Randolph in Chicago and saw his food allergy unit at the Swedish Covenant Hospital. I then tested his method for several years in my general practice at Kew Gardens, and since I became a psychiatrist I have used it on a limited scale at Park Prewett. Joanna's was the first case I had been able to tackle under controlled conditions with as much nursing and ancillary help as I needed. The following letter from Dr Lyon to her GP, written after she had gone home, summarizes the result.

Discharge Report　　　　　　　　Park Prewett Hospital
23 July 1973　　　　　　　　　　　Basingstoke
Dear Doctor

Re: Mrs Joanna D. d.o.b. 2/27/45

This lady has had twelve previous admissions to this hospital. On this occasion she was readmitted on 12 Oct '72 on an informal basis after an attempt to slash her wrists.

She was treated with ECT and a wide variety of medications. Unfortunately she showed little improvement; she remained very tense and there were frequent episodes of self-injury.

On 25 April 1973, she was transferred to the Psychiatric Intensive Care Unit for further assessment. At that time she was extremely tense but quite unable to talk about her problems. Her only resort was either to inflict injury upon herself or to rock persistently like a baby. Under the influence of intravenous

Valium she was able to reveal considerable concern about her relationship with her mother, her own fear that due to masturbation in her youth she was permanently disfigured and her very strong feelings of guilt and unworthiness. She was again fully investigated and the social position reassessed. She was treated with a wide variety of medications in high dosages and she also underwent abreactive treatment. None of this gave any great improvement and eventually she was shown at a case conference with a view to considering a leucotomy.

At this time it was suggested by Dr Mackarness that this could be due to food allergy. In order to inquire into this possibility we set up an experiment in which she was initially starved for five days and then given test doses of specified foodstuffs. The fast resulted in a very marked improvement in her condition and the test doses showed severe reactions to some foods but not to others. As a further test, a trial was undertaken on a double-blind basis. In this test she was given single foods prepared and emulsified with water by the dietitian, their nature being unknown to the nursing staff who gave them via a stomach tube from coded, masked syringes. She rated her own reactions to these feedings and two independent observer ratings were also undertaken. When the code was broken subsequently, it was clear that she had again shown the same severe reactions to the foods previously found to give rise to reactions, and no reactions to the foods found to be 'safe' on open feeding.

During this time her condition had improved so drastically that we were able to discharge her home on no medication at all. Mrs D. knows which foods make her ill and Dr Mackarness has provided her with a menu made up of appropriate safe foods. For your information, I enclose a list of some foods to which she showed a bad reaction and some to which she showed no adverse response. Also enclosed is a copy of the menus suggested by us.*

I must admit that such a remarkable response has been a surprise to me. However, it has been so dramatic that I think it would be difficult for us to say that it was due to anything but the dietary changes, especially in view of the double-blind trial. I

* These items are given in Chapter 5.

hope that her improvement is maintained. Dr Mackarness will follow her up in the Out-Patient Department.

Yours sincerely

J. S. Lyon, MRCP, MRCPsych, DPM Consultant Psychiatrist

Three months later her general practitioner sent me this report:

Since her discharge from hospital in July '73, Joanna has made a remarkable improvement. She is happy, gay, euphoric, sometimes almost hypomanic in her hearty enjoyment of life. She goes out to work, cares for the children without harming them, looks after her house and generally seems to be almost back to her old self before this illness first attacked her.

However, she persistently eats the 'wrong' foods if she wishes to attract attention and sympathy to herself, or to penalize her husband or her doctors; she then rapidly becomes morose, sullen, apathetic and withdrawn, and on one occasion became hallucinated, seeing a herd of deer in a public car park. These attacks subside quite quickly with intramuscular doses of 10 mg diazepam (Valium) and seem to be less frequent as they become less effective in attracting attention.

A year after her discharge from the hospital she had still remained well throughout, apart from three short readmissions when she became ill through breaking her diet. Fasting for two or three days and encouragement to stick strictly to her permitted foods soon got her well again.

Such lapses, in the face of certain knowledge that they will bring the disaster of an acute return of mental symptoms, suggest an addictive element in food and chemical allergy.

The word allergy (literally, other response) was coined in 1906 by Clemens von Pirquet, a Viennese paediatrician who worked on diphtheria in children with Dr Béla Schick, originator of the Schick skin test for immunity to this disease. Von Pirquet defined allergy as an acquired, specific, altered capacity to react to physical substances on the part of the tissues of the body.[24]

Although allergic illnesses have been recognized and described since ancient times, they are still imperfectly understood. It is known, however, that allergies to specific substances are acquired by exposure to those substances and that a general tendency to react in a hypersensitive or allergic manner is hereditary. It has been estimated that a family tendency to allergic reactions affects as much as eighty per cent of the population in developed countries.

Allergy as a medical subject grew up within the frame of immunology: the study of immunity or resistance to infection by the micro-organisms of smallpox, diphtheria, tetanus, typhoid and other contagious diseases. Early researchers in this field found that, in addition to the desirable immune response following the injection of dead germs (called antigens because they generate antibodies), they also encountered hypersensitivity reactions. This discovery led to the development of skin tests for immunity. In such tests a minute quantity of dead germs is injected with a very fine needle into the thickness of the skin. If the patient has had a natural infection with the germ and has overcome it and developed an immunity, redness or swelling will develop around the site of the injection. If there is no immunity, a weal will not appear and the next step is to give a course of more concentrated injections of dead germs until enough protective antibodies have been produced to create immunity and a skin response. These skin tests and subsequent injections form the basis of the public-health immunization programmes established to protect children from such infections as scarlet fever and diphtheria which were responsible for so many deaths in the nineteenth century. However, some people become hypersensitive or allergic as well to the antigens with which they are injected.

Immunity and allergy, the two antithetical responses to inoculation with identical material were explained by von Pirquet as *changed* reactivity following exposure: on the one hand, acquired or induced immunity; on the other, hypersensitivity. Both are based on the chemically understood antigen/antibody reaction and are demonstrable by the skin tests which have since become the *sine qua non* of conventional allergy practice. A patient with hay fever, for example, is subjected to test doses of different pollen extracts injected under the skin, and subsequent immunizing injections are then given against the pollens to which his skin reactions have shown him to be sensitive. In some imperfectly understood way, these immunizing injections boost his resistance to the allergen.

Convention is a powerful force in medicine, and for years now most allergists have restricted their clinical work to conditions like asthma and hay fever which respond to skin tests and desensitizing injections with graded doses of allergens – pollen, house dust and similar inhalant antigens being amongst the most common.

Against this background of almost three-quarters of a century of conventional allergy practice, Albert Rowe in California began drawing medical attention to the importance of food allergy as a factor in many common diseases, and advocating the use of elimination diets as a way of identifying and excluding the foods responsible. His approach was empirical and clinical, in line with von Pirquet's original wide, biological view of allergy.

The idea that food sensitivity could cause mental disturbance was not original with Rowe. In the early 1920s three separate American physicians[13, 23, 36] had drawn attention to changes in the behaviour of children suffering from allergies to food and other substances,* while in France in 1930 Professor Valéry-Radot, doyen of French allergists, reported a case of 'depressive/maniacal reaction' in a patient with food allergy. Rowe, however, pioneered the elimination diet in the treatment of food-allergy symptoms, and he did more than anyone else to bring to world medical attention the wide scope of this dietary treatment, and the variety of chronic symptoms – including mental ones – it could alleviate.

Rowe started work just after the First World War and was an old man when I visited him in 1963. However, he was still active in his practice and showed me over his huge private food-allergy clinic in Oakland, north of San Francisco. His income, he told me, was $193,000 a year after tax! Those patients to whom I talked felt they were getting good value for money.

Some five years earlier, in the winter of 1958, Dr Ted Randolph had shown me several of his patients at the Swedish Covenant Hospital in Chicago. These cases persuaded me that food allergy might be the key to a number of stubborn, puzzling illnesses among patients in my general practice in England.

Like most general practitioners, I had several patients crippled by illnesses for whose symptoms I was unable to find the cause. In the old days it was common practice to tell these people to pull themselves together and hope for the best. Nowadays these illnesses are more often labelled psychosomatic and the patients are offered psychiatric help, although this too may amount eventually to being told to get on with it – in the nicest possible way, of course, and with the prescription of tranquillizing drugs.

* Shannon wrote 'Of particular interest in these cases are the convulsions, indicating a central nervous system involvement, possibly allergic in aetiology.'

If all the time, money and effort spent in hospitals collecting evidence to demonstrate to these people that they have 'nothing physically wrong' with them enabled them to go home cured and reassured, it would be well worth while. In a few cases it does do so, but the majority continue to feel as ill as before, if not worse.

One such patient who consulted me before I made the historic trip to Chicago, was Mrs A., whose story was reported in the July 1959 number of *Medical World*, under the title: 'Stone-Age Diet for Functional Disorders'. She was thirty-two years old, happily married, with one child just starting school. I remember her as a slightly plump, pink-and-white, rather pretty woman, with a soft voice and a house which smelt of furniture polish. She worked as a home help for the Local Authority. She was so pleasant and thoughtful with the old people and invalids she used to visit that she was much in demand.

She attended my surgery, complaining of feeling off-colour and miserable for the past three weeks, with an intermittent pain in the lower abdomen as well. She reported that her 'tummy seemed to puff right out' when she ate, that her periods were becoming heavier, and that she felt easily tired. Examination revealed tenderness in the region of the right ovary.

Three days later she had such an acute attack of pain that I called in the local gynaecologist, thinking that her pain and heavy periods might be connected. He could find no evidence of disease in the pelvis, and blood tests showed only 'very mild iron-deficiency anaemia, white count within normal range'. I reassured Mrs A., gave her iron tablets, and allowed her to go back to work part-time. She was back within a month saying that ever since the gynaecologist's visit she had had intermittent swelling and colicky pain, both of which came on within minutes of eating and would last about two hours. There was no nausea and no diarrhoea; in fact she was rather constipated. She felt well only if she did not eat. I examined her after she had eaten a small meal and could feel a swelling in the vicinity of the appendix.

She was given an antacid mixture containing belladonna to take regularly before meals. Within a week she was back again saying that the mixture made her bowels loose, dried her mouth, and did not relieve the colic or the swelling. By 3 October, nearly two months since she first attended my surgery, she looked really ill and I referred her to the senior surgeon at the hospital for investigation, with a provisional diagnosis of regional ileitis (Crohn's disease).

Barium enema, barium meal and follow-through X-rays were normal and Mrs A. was referred within the hospital to the consultant physician specializing in gastroenterology, who saw her on 20 November. On direct visual examination with the sigmoidoscope he found no abnormality in the rectum or lower colon, and wrote agreeing with my provisional diagnosis, saying it was probably too early for the condition to show on the X-ray.

During the next two weeks Mrs A. had another full blood count which was again normal, and an X-ray of her gall bladder. This, too, proved normal and on 18 December she was discharged home to my care. The gastroenterologist's final report said:

We have failed to find any signs of physical disease in this case, and frankly I doubt if there is any. I talked to her at some length, when I last saw her, about her private life . . . I think that her symptoms are probably related to a period of tension, and as they seem to be settling down now, perhaps further investigation is unnecessary. I have reassured her firmly about her physical state.

By 'tension', this specialist meant emotional tension, a diagnosis frequently applied to people like Mrs A., whose illnesses cannot be explained in terms of orthodox pathology. Since her symptoms had no demonstrable physical basis, the hospital decided that she was not really ill and would get better with firm reassurance. She responded by getting steadily worse. At this point, I left for America.

On my return, I found her much worse. She hadn't felt well enough to work for the past two months and had lost 20 pounds by half-starving herself because of the pain and swelling that came on whenever she had a meal.

I explained to her the ideas I had picked up in America and we decided to try them out. For simplicity I told her to start by eliminating all foods of cereal origin, which had been her staples up to that time. She got herself a child's exercise book and on the first page wrote:

Elimination diet
Avoid all breads, biscuits, cakes and so on made with flour.
Drink only plain water.
Take only one food at a time.
Three meals a day.
If no puff-up [her own words for her abdominal distension], food OK.

I saw her regularly at home in order to go through the exercise book with her, and by the end of the first week we found several foods she could eat without distress: eggs, milk, bacon, red meat and oranges. But bread, potato, canned soups, fish and offal were all bad, white bread being worst of all. White bread was introduced as a test on the fourth day after Mrs A. had been clear of symptoms for two days on non-cereal foods. It resulted in extreme abdominal distension, headache and malaise.

She went on recording her elimination diet for three weeks, occasionally introducing provocative or suspect

30

foods at my suggestion to see whether they made her ill. By the end of that time she was feeling and looking better, had begun to regain weight and was able to return to work. From then until I left Kew five years later, in 1964, she remained well.

Her diet was not too monotonous even at first, as the list of her safe and dangerous foods shows (see tables below). Later we were able to expand it by testing foods she did not normally eat.

Foods causing no reaction

beef, steak	milk, butter, cream
lamb and mutton	coffee, tea
veal	oranges, apples, grapefruit
bacon, ham, pork, chicken	lettuce
eggs	home-made soup (from stock)

Foods causing reaction	*Intensity of reaction*
breakfast cereals	extreme
bread, biscuits, cake	extreme
parsnips	extreme
any frozen vegetable	extreme
jam tart (white flour)	extreme
sausages	extreme
fish	extreme to moderate
potatoes	moderate
Continental sausage	moderate
anything tinned (for example, corned beef, soup, salmon)	moderate
cornflour blancmange	moderate
cheese	slight
beetroot	slight
milk pudding (plus sugar and milk)	slight
tomatoes	slight

Encouraged by the good results obtained with Mrs A., I applied the methods with varying degrees of success to other cases, including patients with 'fibrositis', dizziness, chronic fatigue, obesity, high blood pressure, and asthma. All had physical symptoms for which various 'psycho-somatic' explanations had been given by specialists who had seen them and failed to help them.

In spite of my apparent success I still had a nagging doubt and felt that perhaps the improvements I had been seeing were not the results of dietary and environmental manoeuvres (in some cases I had moved patients exposed to gas to all-electric houses), but were due to suggestion and the contagiousness of my own enthusiasm. However, Michael B. finally removed my doubts on this score.

Seven-year-old Michael B. was the second of three boys, the sons of a hospital engineer and his schoolteacher wife. There was a history of allergic illness (asthma, eczema and ulcerative colitis) on both sides of the family. Michael's father suffered from periodic attacks of disabling giddiness accompanied by nausea and vomiting, which had been diagnosed by a hospital specialist as Ménière's disease.*

Michael was an overactive, red-haired little boy, pleasant and amusing to talk to when he was well. In July 1958, however, before he and his family had joined my list of patients, he had been referred by the school medical officer to a child-guidance clinic because he was becoming increasingly disturbed and hard to manage. His chief troubles were nail-biting, bed-wetting, stammering, insomnia, tremor of the hands, quarrelsomeness and

* A disease caused by congestion of inflammatory or allergic origin in the semicircular canals of the inner ear, which control equilibrium. Among the symptoms are pallor, nausea, giddiness and various transitory disturbances of hearing and vision. It was first described by Prosper Ménière, (1799–1862), a French physician.

inability to concentrate on school work. In his worst phases he would go almost berserk, rushing about smashing his toys and attacking his brothers.

On my return from America in December 1958, his mother came alone to consult me about him for the first time. She was not happy with his progress under child guidance and wondered if anything else could be done. As she was intelligent, I explained the theory of elimination dieting to her and left her to carry it out with Michael without actually seeing him myself. I was anxious to avoid any suggestion that I was using some form of personal influence or psychotherapy on the boy.

He was better within three days of going on a diet which eliminated all processed foods and foods of cereal origin. By the end of the week, when his mother took him for his regular visit to the child-guidance people, he was a normal boy. The psychiatrist, remarking on his improvement, pooh-poohed the idea that the diet had anything to do with it and Michael's mother stopped telling him about it for fear of offending him. She rang me up, worried that Michael's improvement might be no more than coincidence and therefore would not be maintained. I persuaded her to re-introduce all his cereal foods: cornflakes, white bread, iced lollies, biscuits, cakes and milk chocolate. Within two days he was as bad as he had ever been and she telephoned again, in a panic, asking for advice. I told her to put him back on the cereal-free diet. Although she found it difficult to persuade him to give up the carbohydrate to which he seemed addicted, she did succeed after a few days and he became well again.

That was in February 1959. He has remained well ever since, relapsing only when he inadvertently breaks his diet. His mother worked out a fairly full list of foods which

33

cause no reaction, and another of those which bring back his illness.

Foods causing no reaction
all meat, poultry and offal
bacon
eggs
milk
white fish (except skate)
butter
lard
cauliflower
lettuce

cucumber
bananas
apples (non-acid)
oranges (limited)
ice cream (Lyons, Walls or
   Neilsons)
tea
coffee
cocoa

Foods causing reaction	*Intensity of reaction*
wheat flour	extreme
cornflour	extreme
cheese	extreme (especially when cooked)
skate	extreme
herrings	extreme (vomiting)
kippers	extreme (vomiting)
bloaters	extreme (vomiting)
tinned fish	extreme (vomiting)
Marmite	extreme
potatoes	moderate
tinned fruit	moderate
milk chocolate	moderate
cooked tomatoes	moderate
bought sweets (not all)	slight
sharp apples (usually English)	slight
sharp, acid oranges	slight

I could multiply these cases many times from my records. The two I have given are typical and some general conclusions can be drawn from them.

The elimination diet is a straightforward method and

34

its value is demonstrable by cause and effect. Once relief is obtained, the ecological basis of the illness can be proved by re-exposing the patients to the incriminated foods and watching their symptoms reappear.

A study of the lists of food causing adverse reactions in Mrs A. and Michael B. suggests that possibly it is not always the foods themselves that are to blame, but their chemical contaminants. For example, Mrs A. could drink her own home-made soup, but soup from a tin upset her. Soup cans are often lined with a gold-coloured resin to which some people are known to be sensitive. Also, many canned-soup manufacturers add monosodium glutamate, a meaty-tasting flavouring agent which has recently come under fire in the *British Medical Journal* as causing the condition quaintly named Kwok's Quease or the Chinese Restaurant Syndrome.

Dr Robert Kwok is a research investigator practising in America who regularly eats Chinese food. One day, in a Chinese restaurant, he was suddenly seized with the most frightful gripping pain in his chest, running up into his neck. He thought he was going to faint, and more or less collapsed across the table. The acute pain, which he thought was the beginning of a heart attack, subsided after a few minutes, but it left him shaken and determined to find out what had brought on such alarming symptoms. After much research with interested colleagues, he eventually came up with the answer: he had an allergy to monosodium glutamate, which some Chinese chefs add in considerable quantities to the food they prepare. Kwok first published his own case in the *New England Journal of Medicine*[19] and his name and the syndrome associated with it have since become well known to doctors throughout the world.

At the end of my article reporting the cases of Mrs A.

35

and Michael B.,[21] I suggested that allergy to foods and chemicals was a much more common cause of chronic ill-health than most doctors imagined. Here are the concluding paragraphs:

Conclusions

Many theories have been put forward to account for the increase in the number of patients with neurosis and psychosomatic illness today. The psychiatrists have persistently claimed that they have the secret, but somehow they have failed to give the GP a solution he can use.

I do not think we are being subjected to much more psychological stress now than we were twenty-five years ago, but I am sure that the sophistication and adulteration of food with chemical additives has increased enormously in that time and so has the consumption of processed starch and sugar (white bread, cakes, biscuits, sweets and soft drinks).

It would be surprising if people were *not* allergic to pesticides put into the ground and sprayed on crops, to flour 'improvers', anti-staling agents, emulsifying compounds, artificial colourings, preservatives and the whole terrifying array of potentially toxic substances now being added to our food in order to improve its appearance, flavour, shelf-life and profitability.

Why should psychosomatic or functional illness not be a manifestation of allergy to these new synthetic chemicals which we are eating more and more as the supermarkets multiply? I believe the Stone-Age elimination diet to be a means not only of answering this question, but also of giving relief to thousands of people whose health has been affected in this way.

Summary

Food allergy as a cause of disease, particularly the role of processed cereal foods as allergens, is described. An account is given of the treatment of four cases of disabling psychosomatic disorder on non-psychiatric lines, using a Stone-Age (pre-cereal) elimination diet.

The implications of the increasing use of chemical food additives are briefly discussed.

Because ecological illness (food and chemical allergy) is not yet recognized for what it is, no statistical studies have been made, and we can only estimate its incidence. Since I wrote this article, however, I have had much more experience of the subject, and I would now tentatively put the incidence of this type of illness as follows: 30 per cent of people attending GPs have symptoms traceable exclusively to food and chemical allergy; 30 per cent have symptoms partially traceable to this cause, and the remaining 40 per cent have symptoms which are unrelated to allergy. My American colleagues give similar figures. If we are right, there is a need for a complete change in the medical approach to ill-health, and a total revision of government policy and regulations concerning food.

Among the 30 per cent whose symptoms are partially traceable to food or chemical allergy are those in whom the illness is attributable in some degree to psychological factors or conditioning by unpleasant early experiences. Psychotherapy can help such patients and drugs like chlorpromazine which appear to reverse or normalize psychotic (unbalanced) thinking will continue to be needed as long as there is a shortage of psychiatrists and facilities for the overall investigation and care of mental patients. Purely psychological factors are important also in raising or lowering a person's powers of adaptation to stresses of all kinds, of which sensitivity to specific foods and chemicals is but one.

Interestingly enough, Dr John Fry (referred to in the introduction) and his colleagues at the Royal College of General Practitioners in England, who have done careful statistical research into the types of illness dealt with by GPs, have come up with figures very similar to those I have just given — but with regard to emotionally determined illness (or psychosomatic illness, to use the currently fashionable term). Fry estimates that 30 per cent of illnesses are emotionally determined (and he is including depression in this figure) and the rest, with or without an emotional component, are physical or organic in origin: injuries, infections, cancer, degenerative diseases and so on.

Taking Fry's figures and my own as being fairly accurate, the difference in causation can easily be resolved by showing that his 30 per cent supposed to be entirely emotional or psychosomatic (which he says doctors find so mystifying) are really somatopsychic and have an allergic rather than an emotional basis. Identifying and eliminating the foods and chemicals which make these people ill can produce a complete cure in 80 to 90 per cent of the cases. (The earlier the illness is tackled, the more completely reversible is the underlying allergic process.) The remaining 10 to 20 per cent of patients – whose condition is long-standing and in whom oft-repeated allergic reactions have caused irreversible physical changes in the tissues or deeply implanted mental conditioning – can also be helped; but in them the improvement will be only partial, for after many years, pathological changes of a more permanent nature will usually have taken place.

chapter two

Although the ecological lobby in Western countries has been more and more vocal of late, fears have been expressed mainly about the *long-term* effects of chemical additives and contaminants in food, sprays on crops and artificial fertilizers in the soil. Very few people have realized that a lot of us are being made ill *now* by what is being done to the food we eat and the air we breathe. This is because the ecologists and the doctors and scientists who advise them have been thinking in terms of toxicology or poisoning rather than allergy.

In fact, allergy or intolerance to environmental substances is no new thing and has probably always been a by-product of man's evolution in a changing world. The word ecology was first used in 1866[14] to refer to the mutual relations of living things to their physical surroundings and to each other, as described by Darwin. Implicit in the concept of ecological balance is the long and intricate process of adaptation by which men come to live in harmony with their physical environment, and it is a rule of ecology that living creatures show better adaptation to those things to which they have been exposed longest: it is very much rarer to find a patient disabled by eating meat or by normal exposure to sunlight (I am not talking about sunburn), than it is to find one made ill by eating wheat or inhaling the petro-chemicals in the air on a street full of heavy motor traffic.

39

Man's diet has evolved over millions of years, from the monkey-type vegetarian diet of the forest-dwelling gatherers to a carnivorous one. Meat has been man's main food for over nine-tenths of the time since he learned to walk upright and use his hands as tools. Starches and sugars as a basis for nutrition are a very recent introduction: they have been part of our diet for ten thousand years at most, as against two to three million years on meat, fat and protein.

Our modern carbohydrate-based diet of highly refined and processed foods, contaminated by hundreds of newly invented synthetic chemicals, is such a recent innovation that there has not yet been time for extensive study of its effects on man. Most of the evidence beginning to come in, however, suggests that the effects may be harmful.

Living things are distinguished from inanimate objects by their ability to adapt to changes in their environment. 'Adaptation', according to Webster's *New International Dictionary*, is 'modification of an animal or plant (or of its parts or organs), fitting it more perfectly for existence under the conditions of its environment.' 'Modification of an animal' may include structural, functional and behavioural changes, involving the nervous system, the glands and the cellular enzyme system.* In the human organism, the brain and the nervous system have played the major role in determining adaptation and evolutionary progress.

The brain's efficiency depends on the proper working

* Enzyme means, literally, 'in yeast' because the first of them to be described were the ones which live in the mould found on the skins of grapes and turn sugar into alcohol in the fermentation process used in making wine. They are called catalysts because they speed the process of fermentation along. So too, in every cell of the body enzymes speed the processes which give the body its energy and its life.

40

and smooth integration of the other two systems: the endocrine and the cellular enzyme system. The endocrine system consists of the ductless glands, which pour hormones into the bloodstream to regulate the body's functioning. The cellular enzyme, or catalyst, system provides the biochemical reactions by which the brain formulates and transmits messages along the nerve pathways of the body.

The primitive hunter in pursuit of food uses exactly the same nerve signals as the NASA scientist programming the computers which guide a landing on the moon. The difference is only in complexity. In both cases the work is done by the same sort of nervous system built of the same basic materials, chiefly animal fats. No nervous system has ever been built of starch or sugar, and to base a diet on carbohydrates, as millions do today, is to invite the problems of inadequately constructed and malfunctioning brain and nerves.

During the course of his existence, man has had to adapt to many potentially harmful things: heat and cold, wet and drought, injury, infection and change of diet, to mention only a few. As this is a book about food, I shall concentrate on man's adaptation to change in diet, showing how the adaptive process has worked in the past and still works – or fails to work – today.

The adaptation of a species can fail in two different ways: the organism may not be able to reproduce quickly enough to evolve in the face of a new stress; or it may be subjected to unrelieved exposure to too much stress over too long a period.

Failure to adapt for the first reason has occurred down the ages and has led to the disappearance of many species, such as dinosaurs. Problems related to the second reason which are occurring today have been extensively investigated by Professor Hans Selye (pronounced Sel-ee-ay) of Montreal, a pioneer of modern physiological research into stress. Professor Selye defines stress as the struggle to adapt to a noxious agent.

According to one theory, the kind of food available to our remote ancestors determined their evolution from apes to humans. Europe, Asia and Africa were joined together millions of years ago and huge rain forests covered the land. Among the many apes living in this humid jungle were the anthropoids from whom we are descended. Though more or less vegetarian, as the apes are now, living on fruits, nuts, roots, tender shoots and leaves, they also enjoyed eating birds, small animals and fish when they could catch them. Living among the branches of the trees and escaping aloft when danger threatened, these remote ancestors of ours did well as long as the forest flourished.

The climate changed, however, and the land began to dry up. Trees were gradually replaced by open plains and grasslands. As the forests shrank, apes and monkeys were crowded into the dwindling islands of jungle, competing with each other for a diminishing food supply.

Grass-eating animals like deer and horses spread and multiplied as the plains grew, while the apes and their cousins in the trees, lacking the chewing teeth and cellulose-digesting intestines of the herbivores, had either to learn to eat the flesh of those animals or to perish.

Many apes died. The few survivors went on breeding tree-dwelling vegetarians like themselves, as they have continued to do right down to the present day. However, a few of their anthropoid cousins, having more intelligence, came down from the trees and learned to run on two legs, and to hunt and to eat meat. They were the predecessors of modern man.

The difficult transition from tree-dwelling vegetarianism to prairie-running meat-eating was made possible through three gifts: a pair of hands with a thumb opposed to the four fingers; a brain equal to that of a modern four-year-old human child, capable of learning by experience; and time – lots and lots of time. These early hominids had hundreds of generations to acquire by natural selection the adaptive attributes necessary for survival in a changed world.

Darwin's theory of evolution rests on two separate but interdependent processes: mutation and natural selection. When male and female reproductive cells join in the act of conception, the nucleic material which carries hereditary characteristics is juggled about in such a way that the offspring are born unlike their parents in certain respects. This is mutation; occasionally the new altered characteristic is one which can be used to tremendous advantage in the struggle for survival.

A giraffe may be born with a longer neck than its parents, a mutation inherited by chance in the genetic lottery and happening to have great survival value, for the longer-necked giraffe can reach and eat leaves beyond the reach of smaller animals. Similarly, in just the same random way, mutations have helped man to progress beyond his ape-like ancestors. A slight improvement in a part of the nervous system, for instance, could have given better coordination of hand and eye to one of our early ancestors, enabling him to throw his spear more accurately and catch more food. Inheriting his mutation, his children would also be skilled with the spear and able to consolidate their superior position by getting more and better food.

Such mutations help their possessors survive by giving them an advantage over other members of the species in

43

the struggle for existence. The process can also operate in reverse to assure the extinction of maladapted creatures. If a black moth, for instance, produced a white mutant in the sooty, industrial North, the offspring would not have much chance of escaping early consumption by a predatory bird. This is the process that Darwin called natural selection. By it, giraffes' necks have grown longer, men have become cleverer, and moths in sooty areas have got blacker.

Natural selection is a genetic matter: a change in the growth programme of a species cannot be brought about by external alterations of the individual organism. Though generations of 'giraffe-necked' women in Africa have had rings of wire put round their necks to stretch and lengthen them, their children continue to be born with necks of normal length. Dogs who have had their tails docked at birth still produce puppies with long tails.

Biologists believe that it is very rare for a characteristic acquired during a person's lifetime to be inherited, and indeed we still have no firm evidence that it can actually occur.

The smooth operation of mutation and natural selection depends on a continuing supply of suitable food and a reasonably stable physical environment. There is evidence that the elephants in the game reserves of Africa are being wiped out as much by the change in their food supply consequent upon restriction of their normal nomadic way of feeding in the forests as by the activities of illegal ivory hunters. It is quite possible that what we are now doing to food in the industrialized West will produce a similar change so debilitating that we may exterminate ourselves with degenerative diseases or be crushed by a people like the Chinese who handle their food supplies more sensibly.

Time is running out for us; a complete reappraisal of environmental and dietary policies in Europe and America is literally a matter of life and death, and long overdue.

The anthropoids who emerged from the forest onto the prairie were not at first, adept at hunting the big, grass-eating animals and had to live on stray, dead specimens and what they could collect at the edge of the forest: grubs, honey, insects, birds' eggs and small rodents dug out of their burrows. After a time, however, they learned to hide in the grass and pounce on a grazing animal temporarily separated from its herd. Later they worked in packs, as baboons do now, heading off an antelope, pulling it down and killing it. They also learned to throw stones. Thus the anthropoids who moved out onto the grasslands became more and more ingenious in the use of eye, hand and brain. Gradually they grew to look less like apes, more like humans, and they developed a primitive language.

As the grass spread to replace the trees, there was more food to support buffalo, antelope, horses and cattle for men to hunt, and the men themselves became bolder, cleverer and more experienced in hunting. Eventually they invented weapons – clubs, slings and spears – with which to ensure themselves an unlimited supply of life-giving meat. Half a million years ago they discovered fire, which helped them to survive the ice ages.

The painful transition from vegetarian tree-dwelling to carnivorous ground-hunting and cave-dwelling involved serious hardship and a high death rate. Changing from a plentiful diet of leaves and fruit to infrequent meals of meat, marrow and fat surely caused these early humans a lot of indigestion. For a time they must have been less robust than their tree-fed cousins, just as the Icelandic

45

ponies of today, which are forced to live on fish, are poorer specimens than their hay- and corn-fed brothers and sisters in Britain.

These changes took place at least a million years ago, more likely three million. In all these years, according to the palaeontologists who study fossil remains, the true apes have changed little, chimpanzees of today having the same bone-structure and substantially the same vegetarian diet as their ancestors. During the same period the pre-human cousins of the early apes changed profoundly as a result of moving out onto the savannah and becoming meat-eaters. Coming down from the trees was a significant step in the development of human form and intelligence.

One of the more obvious visible changes was the emergence of sharp canine teeth, the pair on either side of the upper incisors, which are useful for meat-eating. In animals which live exclusively on meat like wild dogs and tigers, these teeth are even longer and sharper.

More important, though not appreciated until recent study by biochemists and microbiologists, was the evolution of new metabolic pathways within the cells. These enabled the liver and other tissues to convert animal fats and proteins, instead of the old vegetable foods, into substances which could supply energy to the muscles and other organs. More important still, these new pathways allowed our hominid ancestors to utilize chemical building-blocks, mainly unsaturated fats supplied by the flesh of herbivores, for growing bigger and better brains capable of more (and more effective and imaginative) thought, feeling and behaviour.

The complicated chemical reactions at cell level which enable our bodies and brains to work so marvellously are dependent on a host of enzymes or physiological catalysts which have been perfected through thousands of genera-

46

tions living on natural foods, first wild plants and roots and later free-running fat meat.

Since the late nineteenth century, when the unprecedented wholesale refinement and adulteration of basic foodstuffs began, Western civilization has been increasingly afflicted by a new pattern of epidemic disease: degenerative diseases of the heart, arteries and nervous system have been replacing the infections which swept Europe and America a century ago and against them the products of the pharmaceutical industry try to protect us. When we suddenly confront our meat-adjusted body chemistry with high doses of refined starch, sugar and a host of new, synthetic chemicals, we invite a breakdown in our basic cell processes, of which we are already seeing evidence. It is difficult to realize just how enormously perilous it is to tamper with enzyme systems – the self-lubricating and self-repairing cogs of the body's physiological engine.

Hans Selye will come to rank with Louis Pasteur, Frederick Banting and Alexander Fleming among the immortals of medical research because of his clarification of the mechanics of adaptation and the body's response to the threats to its stability. The object of the research being done in Selye's physiological laboratory at the University of Montreal is to determine the effects on the body of sudden or prolonged exposure to severe stress.

Before going on to describe Selye's work, I need to make it clear that what he means by stress is not the popular conception of the word. Most people think of stress in psychological terms, meaning by 'stressful situations' those which cause nervous tension. Business executives in high-powered companies, labouring under the constant pressure of decision-making, are thought to be particularly susceptible to stress disorders. Yet a person who eats a pre-cereal Stone-Age diet, based on meat, fruit and clean water, and who breathes pure country air is likely to be far better at decision-making or anything else than one who sits in a city office, eats business lunches and inhales the fumes of tobacco and gas heat all day.

Stress, in scientific terms, is the wear and tear induced in the body by the adaptive, day-to-day struggle of the organism to remain normal in the face of potentially harmful agents, including physical and psychological stressors of all kinds, from bad food to noisy neighbours.

Selye has defined stress as the rate at which wear and tear is induced in the body by the process of living. Since some stress is clearly unavoidable, our object must not be to try to avoid stress altogether, but to learn to live with it and minimize its harmful effects. A certain amount of stress is beneficial; it has been recognized since early times that there is a healing force in nature which tends to cure from within, and that this force is activated by stress. Modern research, like Selye's, has helped to clarify and explain the ways in which the body copes with stress. From the work Selye has published so far, it is clear that the mental symptoms that appear when a person is failing to adapt to stress are only one manifestation of the battle of adaptation, and are not themselves the whole disease, as many people believe.

One of the pioneers in the study of stress – some years before Selye – was the late Walter B. Cannon, Professor of Physiology at Harvard University Medical School, who during the late 1920s studied the workings of the autonomic nervous system (those nerves which control automatic functions like digestion, sweating and heartbeat, which cannot ordinarily be influenced by conscious willpower).

He did much of the early work on adrenalin, the 'fight-or-flight' hormone produced by the adrenal glands. In response to the emotions of fear and anger, adrenalin is poured into the bloodstream and carried to every part of the body in a few seconds as a chemical messenger preparing it for immediate, violent action.

Adrenalin makes the heart beat faster, diverts blood from the skin and the bowels to the limb muscles and the brain, dilates the pupils and causes the muscles surrounding the bronchial tubes to relax and let more air into the lungs: all useful preparation for a fight or flight for life.

Cannon coined the word homeostasis (from the Greek (*homeo* = the same and *stasis* = staying) to mean the steady, normal state of the body maintained by the combined actions of adrenalin, the autonomic nervous system and the other adaptive processes which he studied.* Not much was known in his day about the main adaptive hormone, cortisone.

He was fascinated by the paradox of a body composed of soft, perishable materials, yet able to maintain a constant and almost unchanging identity for seventy to eighty years. He put it this way: 'When we consider the extreme instability of our bodily structure, its readiness for disturbance by the slightest application of external forces and the rapid onset of its decomposition as soon as favouring circumstances are withdrawn, its persistence through many decades seems almost a miracle.'[5]

Not only does it seem so, it *is* a miracle – now more than ever, when so many subtle, adverse, external forces are being applied.

* To help his students remember the actions of adrenalin, my old physiology professor R. J. S. MacDowell used to say 'Adrenalin makes a white woman whiter and a dark frog darker.' A white person does go pale with rage or fright, when the tiny blood vessels which give the skin its pink colour are constricted to divert the blood to the muscles; a frog can hide better from its enemies when adrenalin expands the dark patches of pigment in its skin.

Long before Cannon, Hippocrates used the phrase *vis medicatrix naturae* (the healing power of nature) to account for the recovery which took place when the sick body was left to its own devices. One of Hippocrates' aphorisms goes: 'When things are at the crisis, or when they have just passed it, neither move the bowels nor make any innovation in treatment, either as regards purgatives or any other stimulants, but let things alone.'[18] In other words, leave nature to do its wonderful repair work.

Equally sensible and more precise references to the self-regulatory, adaptive powers of the body have been made by the nineteenth-century physiologists quoted by Cannon. The Belgian physiologist, Léon Frédéricq, said in 1885: 'The living being is an agency of such sort that each disturbing influence induces by itself the calling forth of compensatory activity to neutralize or repair the disturbance. The higher in the scale of living beings, the more numerous, the more perfect and the more complicated do these regulatory agencies become.' In 1900, Charles Robert Richet, Professor of Physiology in Paris, took this idea further by drawing attention to the stable instability of the body. 'The living body is stable,' he wrote; 'it must be so in order not to be destroyed, dissolved or disintegrated by the colossal forces which surround it. By an apparent contradiction, it maintains its stability only if it is excitable and capable of modifying itself according to external stimuli and adjusting its responses to stimulation. In a sense it is stable because it is modifiable – the slightest instability is the necessary condition for the true stability of the organism.'

The adrenal glands have two parts: the central medulla, which produces the adrenalin which pours into the blood in response to messages from the brain; and the outer rind or cortex, the function of which was unknown in Cannon's time. We now know that it produces a number of hormones, including cortisone, which keep the body stable in the face of stresses of all kinds. Cortisone serves to counteract allergic reactions, inflammation and damage in general. As hydrocortisone it is included in creams to relieve the irritation of insect bites, where it is more effective than the still-popular antihistamines.

Hans Selye was the first to show, by means of beautifully designed experiments, that hormones from the adrenal cortex, particularly cortisone, are our first protection and our main means of mobilizing the body's defences against allergic reactions and other kinds of disturbance caused by harmful, outside agents.

In 1936, Selye published a historic letter in *Nature*.[38] It began:

Experiments on rats show that if the organism is severely damaged by acute, non-specific noxious agents such as exposure to cold, surgical injury, excessive muscular exercise or intoxications with sub-lethal doses of diverse drugs, a typical syndrome appears, the symptoms of which are independent of the nature of the damaging agent or the pharmacological type of drug employed, and represent rather a response to damage as such.

He went on to describe the three stages of the syndrome he had observed in his rats: *Stage one* comes on six to forty-eight hours after the initial injury. It is characterized by fall in body temperature, loss of muscle tone, low blood pressure, shrinking of the adrenal glands (as they squeeze as much cortisone as possible into the bloodstream in an effort to set things right) and leaking of fluid from the small blood vessels into the tissues. The casualty officer who sets up an intravenous drip for an accident victim is trying to put some of this fluid back and maintain the normal blood volume. Selye's description of stage one corresponds on the whole with what the First Aid people call surgical (as opposed to emotional) shock.

Stage two begins forty-eight hours after the assault on the body's stability. The adrenals greatly enlarge, the oedema or swelling of the tissues begins to subside and cell division ceases. The pituitary, the master gland situated at the base of the brain, produces increased quantities of adrenal-cortex-stimulating hormone (ACTH). When the noxious agent continues to be applied in sub-lethal doses – either as small repeated injuries or as small repeated doses of an allergen or harmful drug – then the rats build up resistance, become adapted to the stress, and apparently return to normal.

At this stage in his experiments, Selye, who was using cold as the stress, tried taking some of his rats out of the cold cage and putting them back into a warm environment for a while before re-exposing them to cold. He found that they had lost their powers of resistance and had to go through the shock reaction of stage one again. If he left the rats in the cold, however, they went on adapting for a long time, apparently growing used to the stress. There seemed no reason why they should not go on indefinitely in this adapted state, once they had got used to it. To his surprise, however, after some weeks in the cold, his rats began to die, one by one, long before their normal life span was reached. They had entered *Stage three*, the stage of exhaustion. Stage three's symptoms were similar to those seen in stage one, but this time there was no stage of resistance or recovery to follow, only death due to exhaustion of the adaptive resources. At post-mortem Selye found the rats' adrenal glands shrunken and wasted, drained of all protective hormones and incapable of producing any more.

Explaining the significance of these three stages, Selye wrote:

We consider the first stage to be the expression of a general alarm of the organism when suddenly confronted with a critical situation, and therefore term it the 'general alarm reaction'. Since the syndrome as a whole seems to represent a generalized effort of the organism to adapt itself to new conditions, it might be termed the 'general adaptation syndrome'. It might be compared to other general defence reactions such as inflammation or the formation of immune bodies.

The symptoms of the alarm reaction are very similar to those of histamine toxicosis or surgical or anaphylactic shock; it is therefore not unlikely that an essential part in the initiation of the syndrome is the liberation of large quantities of histamine or some similar substance, which may be released from the tissues either mechanically in surgical injury, or by other means in other cases. It seems to us that more or less pronounced forms of this three-stage reaction represent the usual response of the organism to stimuli such as temperature changes, drugs, muscular exercise etc, to which habituation or inurement can occur.

Selye's letter occupied less than two columns in *Nature*, and yet it contains the essence of the whole of his work on adaptation. He has spent the last forty years studying stress, using the scientific methods of observation, hypothesis and experiment.* The results have led to enormous advances in medicine and psychiatry: new treatments have been developed for shock, rheumatism and anaphylaxis, and psychiatrists now have a clearer understanding of the physiological basis for nervous breakdown.

Since he is a physiologist and works mainly with animals, Selye has not himself applied his concepts in a clinical setting. If he had, he would have noted – particularly in the field of allergy – that adaptation and maladaptation show themselves more often as specific symptoms related to specific stressors and individuals than as general to all noxious agents and all people. Adolph, Professor of

* For those who would like to read a popular account of Selye's work on stress, I can recommend his book *The Stress of Life*.[35]

Physiology at the University of Rochester School of Medicine, Rochester, New York, observed and reported[1] similar stages of adaptation to those noted by Selye; but he also found that individual animals showed marked differences in their responses to the same agent, and that these responses were more often specific to a particular stress than general to all.

Working with healthy experimental animals, Selye and Adolph exposed them to regular doses of a given harmful material, under controlled conditions, and watched them show alarm, adapt, develop illnesses in the exhaustion stage, and finally die.

Patients do not generally consult their doctors until they are entering the stage of exhaustion in their struggle to adapt to an environmental stress. Lacking a means of turning back the clock in the patient's illness, the doctor is left to speculate on causes and to treat symptoms empirically as they arise.

Thus in psychiatry, in an adaptive case like Joanna's, there is the topsy-turvy situation of one psychiatrist after another mistakenly citing her symptoms as the cause of her illness. Joanna's wrist-slashing was said to be caused by her depression, and her addictive drinking of coffee was attributed to a fixation at the level of oral sexuality. Instead, they should have attributed her entire set of symptoms to the exhaustion caused by constant exposure to foods to which she was allergic.

chapter three

Centuries before the word' allergy was invented, it was known that one man's meat could be another man's poison, and great variations in people's responses to the same foods were reported in the earliest medical records. But, until recently, abnormal sensitivity to specific foods has been regarded more as a curiosity than a phenomenon worth studying. It was not until around 1925 that some allergists began to suspect that day-in, day-out exposure to certain common foods might be causing chronic illness on a wide scale.

It is easy to accept as allergic the rash which appears when a susceptible person eats shellfish or strawberries, but harder to recognize that the bread or eggs he eats every day may be causing his bouts of catarrh, headache and mental depression. Early reports of allergic reactions to foods were concerned only with immediate, clear-cut cause-and-effect responses to uncommon and rarely eaten foods. Acute reactions to inhaled substances like dust and feathers were also readily accepted as allergic.

A hundred years ago, an ear, nose and throat surgeon named William Harvey* designed an elimination diet for William Banting, a fashionable London undertaker, who had consulted him about his deafness. Harvey prescribed a diet which cured not only his deafness, but also his obesity

* No relation to the famous Harvey who first described the circulation of the blood.

55

(Banting had been terribly fat) and a number of other chronic ailments he had borne with fortitude for many years.

Harvey's diet excluded all foods of cereal origin, but allowed unlimited quantities of fat meat and a good deal of alcohol, on the theory that 'starch and saccharine matter tended to create fat'. 'Quantity of diet may safely be left to the natural appetite,' wrote Banting in his delightful little book on the subject.[3] 'It is quality only which is essential to abate and cure corpulence.' Banting's deafness cleared up when he lost weight because, as Harvey had suspected from the first, the deposits of fat in the openings to his ears had sealed off his eardrums, preventing the sound from reaching them.

This high-fat, high-protein diet, which Banting published in 1864 as a cure for obesity, was opposed by the doctors of that time and criticized as being 'freakish and unscientific'. However, it was successful with the public, and Banting's name passed into the language as a synonym for dieting. I can just remember my grandmother saying that she was banting when she meant she was trying to lose weight.

It remained for medical pioneers like Shannon, an American paediatrician, and Francis Hare, an Australian psychiatrist who ran a clinic for alcoholics at Beckenham in Kent, to point out in the early part of this century that daily exposure to common foods could cause and maintain chronic symptoms. Shannon excluded eggs at one time, and wheat at another, from the diet of disturbed and sick children;[36] and Hare in his mammoth two-volume work *The Food Factor in Disease*[16] gave numerous case histories to support his hypothesis that many common ailments could be caused by a constitutional inability to metabolize starches and sugars properly.

Notwithstanding this early work, little came of these ideas until 1926, when Albert Rowe published his first observations on elimination dieting which he later amplified in *Clinical Allergy* (1937).[31]

It is now some fifty years since Rowe first used his elimination diets to prove that chronic ailments like migraine, dyspepsia, eczema and ulcerative colitis could be cleared up by eliminating wheat, eggs, milk and other common foods from patients' diets. Rowe and others, notably Professor Truelove of Oxford,[37] have shown that the elimination of milk and milk products can cure at least one case in five of ulcerative colitis, a crippling disease of the large bowel which can lead to cancer. Nevertheless, in some of our hospitals, ulcerative colitis is still being treated with bland diets based on milk, with psychotherapy, steroid hormones, and, most drastically, by surgical removal of the large bowel followed by colostomy (construction of an artificial anus in the abdominal wall). It is difficult for anyone who has not undergone a colostomy or had to live with someone who has, to imagine the situation in all its gruesome detail: the smell, the inconvenience of having to change the waste bags, the constant effort to prevent inflammation of the skin around the stoma (the opening in the abdominal wall through which the patient now defecates), and finally the devastating effect it has on the victim's sex life, not to mention his or her general self-confidence.

Rowe distinguished in his work between immediate and delayed reactions to foods. He did not discover, however, that what would ordinarily be a delayed reaction could be converted into an immediate one for diagnostic purposes. A regular food is eliminated from the patient's diet for four or five days and is then given to the patient again, on a test basis. If allergy exists, the symptoms will return within a matter of minutes, or perhaps an hour, in acute and easily recognizable form. This procedure, established by Dr Herbert Rinkel, made it possible for chronic, 'masked' food allergy to be easily identified and verified.

Immediate or acute allergy is recognized and accepted by most people: the swelling of the lips after a mouthful of lobster, for instance, or the red and smarting eyelids some women suffer from when they use certain brands of mascara. Although this type of allergy is common, it is actually far less common than delayed, chronic or, in Rinkel's term, 'masked' allergy. In this type of allergy, the victim actually feels *better immediately after exposure* and symptoms connected with the allergy may be delayed for two or three days. Not surprisingly the food or substance responsible is rarely suspected: if it is a well-liked food, the victim goes on eating it daily in the mistaken belief that it must be good for him because he feels good when he eats it.

Rinkel stumbled on the diagnostic procedure for unmasking hidden allergies quite accidentally, in the course of experiments with his own diet designed to uncover a cure for the chronic catarrh, fatigue and headache which afflicted him.

Rinkel was a large man, a former football full-back, who had gone into the First World War at the age of eighteen as a regimental photographer. Though he was married and had a son and no money by the time he came out of the army, he refused to be deterred from going to medical school. For the next four years he lived almost exclusively on eggs, which his Kansas farmer father sent him, a case at a time, to help save money on his food.

During those four years he became progressively more ill, with a continually running nose and many sore throats and ear complications. By his own account, his catarrh was exceptionally severe. When he had his hands in the sink developing films and did not want to interrupt what he was doing, he would let his head drop between his outstretched arms and the ropes of mucus running from his nostrils would join and touch the floor.

In spite of this disability, he graduated first in his class at Northwestern University Medical School in Illinois, and opened a practice in a large town fifty miles from Chicago. There Rinkel read Rowe's work and decided to experiment with his own diet to see if food allergy was to blame for his nasal symptoms. One day he ate six eggs as quickly as possible, thinking that if he was egg-sensitive he would get an acute reaction. But nothing happened. On the contrary, he felt better than usual. It was not until four years later, when he had moved to Oklahoma City and was studying allergy, that he tried eliminating eggs, which he still liked and ate daily, to see if that would stop his headache, fatigue and running nose. This was the first time since he started medical school that he had ever been without eggs, even for a day.

He found that after two or three days without eggs, he felt better. On the fifth day he ate a piece of birthday cake his wife had made him, not realizing there was egg in it. Ten minutes later he collapsed on the floor in a dead faint and did not come round for several minutes. Rinkel concluded that he must have been acutely sensitive to something in the cake, so he asked his wife about the ingredients. She told him the cake contained, among other things, three eggs.

He reasoned that his five days without eggs had made him highly sensitive to them, so that even the small amount in the slice of cake had caused an acute allergic reaction.

59

Working on this theory, he stayed off eggs for another five days. On the fifth day he ate an egg and suffered another equally acute reaction.

Rinkel then began checking patients at his allergy clinic in Oklahoma City, taking them off certain foods completely and watching for acute reactions when he fed them the food again after five to seven days. He thus worked out a method of testing for masked food sensitivity, which he wrote up and submitted to the American *Annals of Allergy*. The article was promptly rejected. Rinkel was so angry that he decided he must work out his method to the very last detail before again submitting an account of it for publication.

He worked on his theory for eight years, during which time he performed over twenty thousand individual food tests on patients. He presented his results in 1941 before the Southwest Allergy Forum, Fort Worth, Texas, and again in 1944 at a meeting of the Doctors' Diners Club in Oklahoma City where he met Ted Randolph for the first time. The report was subsequently published in 1944.[28]

Since the concept of masking is essential to the understanding of chronic allergic illness, it is well worth taking a bit more time to make this extraordinary phenomenon clear. Rinkel defined masking thus: 'If one uses a food every day or so, one may be allergic to it but never suspect it as a cause of symptoms. It is common to feel better after the meal at which the food is used than before mealtime. This is called masked food allergy.' In other words, masking is the reduction or eradication of symptoms as a result of eating, within a specified time period (generally up to three days), the very food to which the patient originally reacted. Rinkel did not know why the symptoms were abated in this way. He simply observed that it happened.

60

Various modifications of Rinkel's technique can be used to unmask hidden food allergy. In my general practice I used the following procedure: the patient is first questioned about symptoms and food habits. If the symptoms fluctuate and they resemble those seen in food allergy, regularly eaten common foods are suspected and avoided for four to five days. This is best done by fasting, but if the patient cannot take time off work, this fast can be replaced by a diet of meat and water only. Allergy to plain meat is very rare, because we have been well adapted to it for so many millions of years. Water intake is encouraged. On the first and second days salts * are taken in the water to encourage bowel movement and rid the body of trouble-causing foods still in the intestine.

If masked food allergy is the cause of the symptoms, there will be great improvement by the fourth day. When time allows, the fast is continued for one more day to stabilize the patient in a symptom-free state.

Single feedings of each of the avoided foods are then given. Those to which there is no susceptibility will cause no reaction. Others will induce sharp reactions within minutes, or an hour or two at most.

The most striking thing about this unmasking of food allergies is the satisfaction with which patients suddenly recognize their old, familiar symptoms for what they are: simple physical reactions to the food they have been eating. One intelligent woman who suffered from nasal allergy, fatigue and disabling mental depression remarked what a wonderful relief it was to know that her tiredness and miserable self-accusation could be switched off by avoiding eggs and milk – and switched on again by eating them. It

* Epsom salts (magnesium sulphate) will do, or mix two parts sodium bicarbonate with one part potassium bicarbonate, and take a tablespoon in half a pint of warm water, well stirred.

is heartening to know the cause of an illness and be able to do something about it, instead of wondering whether you are a freak or going insane. To know, in fact, that it is *not* all in your mind.

The next important contributor to the understanding of food allergy is the late Dr Arthur Coca, founder of the respected American *Journal of Immunology*. He was professor of Pharmacology at Cornell Medical Center until he became medical director of the Lederle Company, which later amalgamated with the Cyanamid Company (both well-known US pharmaceutical firms).

While he was at Lederle, Coca noticed that his wife, who had been in charge of the experimental animals at Cornell, was not eating certain foods any more, and asked her why. She said that when she ate these foods her pulse raced unpleasantly – up to 160 beats per minute. He confirmed these pulse changes in her and noted a similar pulse acceleration in himself. From these observations, Coca developed the pulse acceleration test as a diagnostic procedure to test for food allergy. His first book on the subject, *Familial Nonreaginic Food-Allergy*, was published in 1942.[7]

The pulse test is not entirely reliable, but I have found it to be a helpful diagnostic aid when used in conjunction with planned avoidance of specific foods. It has the merit of great simplicity and patients can be taught to use it themselves in determining their own allergies.

Far and away the most influential man in researching the subject of food and chemical allergy is Theron (Ted) Randolph MD of Chicago, to whom I have dedicated this book.

At one time an instructor in medicine at Northwestern University, Randolph later practised internal medicine, with a special interest in allergy, in and around Chicago. He knew Albert Rowe well and first met Herbert Rinkel in 1944 at the meeting where he presented the results of his work on masked food allergies. Randolph confirmed Rinkel's findings in his own practice.

I first met Randolph in 1958, when I stayed with him and his wife Tudy in Chicago and saw the work he was doing in his food allergy unit at the Swedish Covenant Hospital.

Ted Randolph is tall and slightly stooped, with a thin face and glasses, suggesting a lanky, benevolent bird, or that most endearing of American actors, James Stewart. I have never known a more single-minded man, nor a doctor who took such immense trouble with his patients. In relation to the time he puts in, his fees are modest by US standards and he never gives a patient up as hopeless. Not surprisingly, his patients love him.

Randolph heard Selye present his new concept of the general adaptation syndrome in 1944,[34] at an allergy society meeting, eight years after his famous letter appeared in *Nature*. But it was not until 1954, ten years later, that Randolph realized that Selye's three stages of adaptation – alarm (non-adapted and immediately reactive), resistance (adapting) and exhaustion (again non-adapted) – explained the phenomenon of masking which he, Rinkel and an allergist named Zeller had written up together in their book *Food Allergy*, published in 1951.[26]

The best way to explain Randolph's application of Selye's three stages of adaptation is in terms of addiction (which I believe to be a form of allergy).

The addict goes through three distinct stages of adaptation to his 'poison', whether it be the whisky of the alcoholic, the bread or sugar of the carboholic (carbohydrate addict) or the glue- of the glue-sniffer. Allergy rarely exists from the beginning. Usually it arises as a result of repeated, widely spaced doses of the potentially harmful substance. Once allergy is established, each widely spaced contact with the offending substance will give a sharp and immediately unpleasant reaction. This is stage one, the stage of alarm, in which the person is non-adapted and reacts at once. The whisky drinker finds that he cannot drink without feeling groggy and ill. The carbohydrate-sensitive person experiences bloating and abdominal discomfort soon after eating a slice of bread, and the petrol- or glue-sniffer gets a nasty headache after each sniff. But this stage is short-lived. If the potential addict increases the frequency of his dose, taking it daily or more often, *a change in the timing of the reaction takes place -* each oft-repeated dose is now followed by a feeling of buoyant well-being rather than the previous malaise. If the regular daily or twice-daily dose is omitted for two or three days, however, the addict (for he is now addicted) will on his resumption experience again the disabling, hangover-like symptoms that used to be his immediate reaction. Naturally, he soon learns to resort more and more frequently to the substance which seems to pick him up and keep him feeling well as long as he consumes it often enough. If he continues to take regular, frequent doses, he will, depending on the strength of his adaptive responses, be able to continue feeling alert and energetic for months or years.

Clinical examples make this clearer. Take the alcohol addict first. A girl was engaged to a man who liked going to pubs and drinking beer. They went together every weekend and she dutifully drank her beer, occasionally going out to the cloakroom to vomit because she found it nauseated her. Gradually, because she was very fond of her

64

boyfriend, she began to drink beer with him more often, occasionally meeting him at lunchtime to do so. Soon, to her astonishment, the beer began to agree with her and her reputation as a hard-headed drinker grew, greatly pleasing her fiancé. How and why she became an alcoholic I shall explain later.

Another example: the petrol-, glue- or paint-sniffer. While I was in general practice, I used to employ a painter, whom I will call Joe, to do decorating jobs in the evening. Since he worked for a local firm of painters during the day, he was never far from an open can of paint. Though he seldom took a holiday, one year he decided to spend a week in Brighton.

Soon after getting down there, on about the second day of his holiday, he began to feel a baffling inner tension and discomfort and a craving for the smell of paint. Walking on the seafront waiting for the pubs to open, he saw a painter working on the ironwork of the pier and immediately struck up a conversation with him, gratefully inhaling huge lungfuls of air heavy with paint fumes. He felt better at once and for the rest of his holiday spent many hours with his new friend, breathing in the paint.

Joe's behaviour was quite automatic. He had no idea why he was so glad to talk to the painter on the pier nor why it made him feel better. He was, of course, topping himself up with regular doses of his addictant to keep himself alert, adapted and in Selye's stage two.

Years later, as his powers of adaptation to paint fumes tailed off and he moved into stage three, the stage of exhaustion, he found that paint no longer picked him up, but made him feel ill. He began to take more and more time off from work, his standards fell and he became slovenly and careless, resorting more and more to beer to damp down his symptoms and keep him going. When I last saw him he was heavily addicted to beer and working only intermittently. The cure would have been to change into a job involving no contact with paint fumes and to stop drinking.

The beer-drinking girl followed a similar path. As she strove to maintain the liveliness which came with every drink of beer and to avoid the hangover symptoms which accompanied abstinence, she became a compulsive drinker. When her adaptation was exhausted she entered stage three – she became ill, with vomiting and headaches following every drink. She had 'lost her tolerance for drink' as the experts in alcoholism put it, for this is a well-known stage in the alcoholic's progress to perdition. Fortunately, at this point she sought medical help. The boyfriend who had started her on beer, now her husband, proved most understanding. With his help she was persuaded to enter a treatment unit for alcoholics and eventually, by abstaining from beer and participating in group therapy, she achieved contented sobriety and became a pillar of the local Alcoholics Anonymous.

Eventually, in addiction, the adaptation to a specific harmful substance (food, drink or chemical) runs out, just as it did for Selye's rats in the general adaptation syndrome. The victim of the addiction has to resort to larger and more frequent doses in order to remain out of the hangover zone, which is entered more and more often and lasts longer and longer as time goes on and the powers of adaptation begin to run out. This is the beginning of stage three, the stage of exhaustion, where again unpleasant hangover reactions follow close on every exposure and come to occupy more and more of the day. In most cases, this is regarded by doctor and patient as the beginning of the illness. The alcoholic drinks before breakfast to relieve hangovers which make the morning unbearable, while the tobacco addict chain-smokes and hoards cigarettes 'in case I run out'. The food addict has biscuits or chocolate by the bedside to relieve the sinking feeling he gets with the onset of a hangover from sugar or starch withdrawal during the night.

In all cases, while the victim is still in stage two and resorting ever more frequently to the 'hair of the dog' to keep feeling well, giving up the addictant will put him back in the non-adapted, immediately susceptible state of stage one, the stage of alarm.

Hangover symptoms take four or five days to clear up (and in the firmly addicted alcoholic they may take the form of delirium tremens or convulsions). When the patient is feeling well again, re-exposure to the 'poison' will bring on a sharp, immediately recognizable recurrence of unpleasant symptoms – thus clearly establishing their cause.

Tobacco, dust, pollen, spores, hair, animal dander and other particles produce minor reactions: greater effects are seen with foods, food-derived alcoholic drinks, drugs, odours, fumes and such chemical emanations as coal gas and petrol-engine hydrocarbons.

Four hundred years BC, Hippocrates recognized the addictive nature of food allergy when he observed: 'There are certain persons who cannot readily change their diet with impunity; and if they make any alteration in it for one day, or even for a part of a day, are greatly injured thereby.'[18] He was describing the hangover effects of withdrawal from a frequently eaten food to which susceptibility exists. The withdrawal effect – an accentuation of chronic reactions when frequently eaten allergenic foods are suddenly avoided – is a cardinal feature of adaptive illness. Understanding of it is vital.

The individual food ingestion test developed by Rinkel

was used on out-patients and did not involve starvation, but only the complete elimination of a formerly regularly eaten food to which the patient was suspected of having a masked allergy. The suspected food was avoided until the patient's absence of symptoms demonstrated that the effects of his last dose had worn off and he had fully recovered from all withdrawal symptoms. Test re-exposure to the suspected food then induced an acute reaction in which cause and effect were obvious. Thus the food allergy was unmasked.

Randolph refined Rinkel's technique by taking his patients into a hospital ward specially screened against all possible allergens and having them fast for five days on nothing but spring water. He then tested them with foods known not to have been either sprayed or processed with chemicals. In this way he was able not only to increase the sharpness of the test response, but also to distinguish between allergy to the foods themselves and allergy to the chemical additives and contaminants.

Chemicals in the diet, which are eaten every day, are not suspected of causing allergic illness even by those most alarmed by their use. Poisoning, not allergy, is what is feared.

Randolph, however, says in his book *Human Ecology and Susceptibility to the Chemical Environment*[27] that he has found chemical additives and contaminants of air, food, water and chemically derived drugs to be a commoner cause of allergy and chronic illness than the more generally recognized naturally occurring physical and biological materials, such as unprocessed foods, animal products and plants. He has demonstrated that one-third of his patients have major allergies to new materials in the chemical environment. For another third, such allergies, while not 'major',

68

appear to be a significant contributing factor to their problems. Randolph's demonstration of the role these new allergens play in the production of the symptoms now afflicting so many people in civilized countries is his most important contribution to medicine.

The following case, taken from his book on chemical susceptibility, is a good illustration of his findings.

Mrs N. R., housewife, age thirty-one, was first seen because of repeated bouts of rhinitis, fatigue, headache, myalgia and low-grade temperature elevations suggestive of influenza. She also complained of being dopey, groggy, unable to read comprehendingly or to think clearly. When these symptoms were intensified she was unusually depressed. At other times she was irritable, unsteady on her feet and frequently dropped things.

She was found to be highly sensitive to several common foods. Although she profited by their avoidance, she remained chronically sick. The fact that she was better during summer months and on vacations when away from home – also the fact that the symptoms recurred soon after she returned home – suggested susceptibility to house dust or indoor chemical air pollution. Although she was found skin-test-sensitive to house dust and knew that dust exposure accentuated her rhinitis, treatment at various levels with house dust extract did not afford satisfactory relief.

Her chronic symptoms during winter months were at least 50 per cent improved following the simultaneous elimination of her gas range, gas refrigerator and gas water-heater from her kitchen, and substitution of electrical equipment . . .

With the control of indoor air pollution, the avoidance of major chemically contaminated foods, and a few other specific susceptibilities, this patient has remained well.

The allergic effect of gas and petrol fumes is difficult to place in terms of what is known as immunology, which allergists invoke to try to explain all types of allergy, but it has been pointed out by other allergists* that certain highly susceptible people are made ill by exposure to such substances, even in minute dosage.

Keeping patients like Mrs N. R. symptom-free may involve such a vast restructuring of home, working conditions and eating habits that they will undertake it only when they have been seriously ill for a long time and are utterly convinced of the soundness of the ecological approach. Over the last ten years, more than two thousand of Randolph's patients in and around Chicago have been sufficiently convinced to remove all gas-burning appliances from their houses in order to remain well.

While he was working out his patients' reactions to indoor and outdoor air pollution, Randolph was also establishing the importance of chemical additives and food contaminants in specific adaptive illness.

He worked out the following system for testing the effects of such contaminants. First he gave his patients uncontaminated forms of all the foods they normally ate at least once every three days. This was to establish that they were not allergic to the foods themselves. Then, three times a day for at least two days, he gave them testfeedings of seldom-eaten safe foods containing additives and/or contaminants. He chose commercially marketed foods known to be contaminated with crop sprays and chemicals added in processing – pesticides, fungicides, sulphur dioxide and other preservatives, artificial colourings, resins used in can linings and so on. The foods chosen were canned peaches, canned dark red cherries, canned salmon, canned tuna, frozen broccoli, frozen cauliflower, frozen spinach, raw apple, raw celery and the outside

* Brown in 1949, and Brown and Colombo in 1954[4] reported on patients who developed bronchospasm from the odours and fumes from oil-burning cooking stoves.

leaves of lettuce. For each contaminated food he used, its pure equivalent was available to be used as a control. If a patient reacted to frozen broccoli spears but was unaffected by those brought fresh from an organic farm, then the chemical contaminants, not the broccoli itself, were suspected.

He found that extremely susceptible patients showed acute reactions following the first ingestion of a chemically contaminated food (after the usual five-day avoidance) but less susceptible patients needed two or more days' cumulative ingestion before they showed convincing symptoms of reaction. Randolph emphasized that allergy to the foods themselves and to their chemical contaminants can give rise to identical symptoms, although those associated with the latter tend to be more severe.

His discovery and clinical exploration of this aspect of allergic disease led Randolph, in the early '50s, to seek out sources of unsprayed, compost-grown food for his patients. He eventually found a farmer west of Chicago who could provide regular supplies of meat untreated with antibiotics and fly sprays, and fruits and vegetables grown without chemical fertilizers or pesticides. Randolph's work has given fresh impetus to the 'health food' movement and provides medical backing for the growing demand for organically grown, pesticide-free foods.

part two

chapter four

In 1937, Albert Rowe said, 'Allergy, next to infection, is probably the most common cause of human symptomatology.' Sir James Mackenzie* (1853–1925), one of the greatest clinicians of all time, admitted towards the end of his life that in three out of four cases he was unable to make a diagnosis. Warning against the complexities brought about by extensive specialization in medicine, Mackenzie wrote, 'For the intelligent practice of medicine and the understanding of disease, the simplification of medicine is necessary . . . I hold the view that the phenomena which at present are so difficult of comprehension on account of their number and diversity are all produced in a few simple ways, and that with their recognition what is now so complex and difficult will become simplified and easy to understand.'

Doctors readily accept this idea of a single basic disease process when dealing with infection. Why not also with allergy and specific adaptation?

Infection with any germ may affect different parts of the body in different ways. The pneumococcus microbe, for example, will produce the clinical signs of pneumonia

---

* Mackenzie started out as a general practitioner in Burnley, Lancashire, and later became a celebrated London heart specialist. His classical book *The Study of the Pulse* (published in 1902) was based on original observations he had made as a GP. Mackenzie invented the ink polygraph, the forerunner of the modern electrocardiograph.

75

when growing in the lungs, and the symptoms of meningitis when growing on the membranes of the brain. The important thing is to make the diagnosis of pneumococcal infection and to get after the germ with an antibiotic to which it will respond.

So too with allergy. Though we may not yet know why some people are more susceptible to allergy than others, nor why the allergic 'target organ' is the gut in one patient and the nervous system in another, it is enough to realize that a set of symptoms may be allergic, and to identify and remove the allergenic substance or, if that is impossible, to strengthen the patient's powers of adaptation to it.

I myself believe that specific adaptive disease is a widespread cause of chronic ill-health in many people and that at least as much should be known about it as is known about infection. It should be taught as a major subject to medical students right at the beginning of their clinical career so that they think of it as a possibility in every patient they see. Dr William Duke, another pioneer American allergist, foresaw the significance of specific adaptive illness in his book *Allergy*, published in 1927[18], when he wrote:

In specific hypersensitiveness, we have a subject which deals with illnesses caused by inert matter. It is nevertheless as broad and may prove as important as the illnesses caused by living matter, that is, bacteria.

Wilder Penfield, the Canadian neurosurgeon and neurophysiologist, has shown that experimental irritation of small, circumscribed areas on the surface of the brain will evoke the same memories and emotional responses in the same subject whenever the stimulus is applied at that particular spot. If an electrode carrying a weak electric current – such as that used by Penfield – has this specific effect time after time, then a localized allergic reaction, involving as it does swelling, lack of oxygen and chemical irritation, may be expected to have a similar, repeatable effect whenever a specific area of brain cells is involved.

Allergists know that every allergic person has his or her special 'target organs', areas of the body which tend to be involved in allergic reactions time after time. In one person it will be a particular patch of skin, in another the lining of the nose or gut, and in a third it will be an area of brain tissue. If this piece of brain tissue happens to be in the part of the brain responsible for muscular movement, the manifestation of the allergy may be an epileptic seizure. Randolph has a film of a wheat-sensitive patient who had fits every time wheat was fed to her, while other foods, to which she was not allergic, had no such effect. If the part of the brain affected is one that controls certain behaviour patterns, then allergic irritation will produce recognizable mental or behavioural changes – changes which may be repeated whenever that particular allergen is applied to that particular person. All allergic people tend to show specific responses to specific substances, rather than general responses to all allergens indiscriminately. This specificity – a particular response by a particular person to a particular stressor – is a fact of life and the one thing above all others which enables doctors to recognize, classify and correctly treat illnesses.

The general tendency to become allergic or sensitized to foreign substances is an inherited characteristic. If you have allergic parents and grandparents, you will probably develop some allergy yourself. But the *kind* of allergy and the *substance* to which you are allergic will be peculiar to yourself and will depend on several things. In food allergy, it will be influenced by the amount you eat of the food in question and how often you eat it; also on the degree to which you are susceptible to that food (i.e. the extent to which it picks you up and lets you down) as well as the power that the food has to sensitize people in general.

Whether you actually develop symptoms when you eat that food, and how bad the symptoms are, will depend on the state of your adaptive defences at the time. You are more likely to react if you have been fighting off a cold and have had an emotional struggle with a loved one than if you are in robust health, happy and settled.

The idea that emotional factors can influence allergy has come to be widely accepted. But most people assume that the emotion causes the allergy, whereas I believe that the emotion causes only an exhaustion of protective hormones, thus lowering the defences against allergy to a substance that otherwise might not cause much trouble.

Foster Kennedy, a Scottish neurologist who worked in America and was interested in allergy and the nervous system, taught that emotion could trigger off an allergic reaction, but he never said, as some psychiatrists do, that one *caused* the other. Kennedy drew an analogy between the allergic skin rash called urticaria or hives (in which there is a patch of swelling) and migraine, a violent headache confined to one side in which there is a swelling of blood vessels at the temple and of the brain membrane nearby. He suggested that local allergic swelling was the common factor in the two illnesses. It is interesting that more and more doctors are beginning to point to food allergy as a major cause of migraine.

It is important to keep in mind that in specific adaptive illness we are dealing with a reversible *process* with recognizable stages, not an irreversible change demonstrable only in the pathology laboratory or on the post-mortem table. When confronted with easily recognizable symptom complexes like high blood pressure, duodenal ulcer and asthma, all of which may appear during the course of an

78

allergic disease, doctors will generally either accept the symptoms as allergic, or label them with words like 'functional', 'idiopathic', 'psychosomatic' or 'essential' – mere cover-ups for uncertainty. We must not allow such symptoms to blind us to the underlying three-stage adaptive process which may be going on. On the contrary, once we have ascertained the sets of symptoms commonly associated with specific adaptive illness, we can see them as indications of this underlying process.

A person with variable chronic symptoms, the causes of which have never been found, is quite likely to be a casualty of the battle of specific adaptation. Evidence of more than one symptom from the following list makes the diagnosis probable. Three or more make it certain. Of course, there are other causes for these symptoms, such as infection or degeneration, which may coexist with allergy. *But in every case where a specific adaptive process is going on, the identification and elimination or neutralization of causative physical materials is necessary before complete relief of symptoms can be obtained.* The following five general symptoms are of particular importance, and these symptoms must fluctuate.

1 Persistent fatigue, not helped by rest
2 Over- or under-weight, or a history of
   fluctuating weight
3 Occasional puffiness of face, hands, abdomen and ankles
4 Palpitations, particularly after food
5 Excessive sweating, unrelated to exercise

At least one of these symptoms is invariably present in all patients with specific adaptive illness. In addition, one or more of the following chronic local symptoms will be present, depending on the part of the body involved in the specific allergic reaction. (Other possible causes, such as infection and injury, for the conditions listed must, of course, be considered, since allergy is the great mimic in medicine.)

Respiratory system

Conjunctivitis Red eyes. The conjunctiva, or covering membrane of the surface of the eye, is continuous with the mucous membrane of the nose, via the lachrymal ducts.

Rhinitis Running or blocked nose, often referred to as catarrh. Not the same as the common cold. May be perennial or intermittent. Includes 'hay fever', which is neither a fever nor often due to hay. Most doctors now call hay fever 'allergic rhinitis'.

Bronchitis The allergic element in this disease is not as well recognized as the infective factor. Tobacco allergy is frequently implicated: so is allergy to petrochemical fumes.

Asthma Sensitivities to foods and chemicals are as important as those to inhalant allergens. Emotional factors can act as a trigger by lowering general resistance, particularly in asthma because respiratory changes are often associated with fear.

Skin

Pruritus Itching, with or without an accompanying rash. Pruritus is common around the anus and the genitals.

Eczema Particularly in infants and children. Milk and woollen clothes are often to blame.

Urticaria White or red raised weals on the skin, usually itchy. Widely recognized as being allergic in origin.

Dermatoses Various eruptions due to direct contact with irritants like nickel and perfume, or to drugs taken orally (e.g. aspirin, phenacetin, penicillin) and to their colourings and flavourings.*

* See the work of Ben Feingold on colouring and flavouring agents in *Why Your Child Is Hyperactive*.[14]

Digestive system

Aphthous ulcers Ulcers which appear inside the mouth and on the tongue; they can be painful and slow to heal.

Dyspepsia Including abdominal distress generally, particularly flatulence and 'bloating'.

Peptic ulcer Including gastric and duodenal ulcer symptoms (often without demonstrable ulcer crater on barium X-ray).

Regional ileitis (Crohn's disease) Inflammation and spasm of the small intestine; ulceration around the anus.

Constipation and diarrhoea Usually allergic in origin when there is no apparent cause.

Colitis Including mucous colitis and ulcerative colitis, the irritable colon syndrome and colic.

Cardiovascular system

Abnormal pulse rhythm Including unusually slow or unusually rapid heartbeat (palpitations).

Anginal pain Pain in the left side of the chest without ischaemic heart disease.

High blood pressure Usually allergic in origin when there is no arteriosclerosis or kidney disease.

Spasms of arteries in the extremities Leading to cramps, chilblains, and inability to exercise without pain. Allergic in origin when there are no accompanying pathological changes in the arteries.

Vasovagal attacks Periodic fainting fits and attacks of feeling unwell all over and having to sit or lie down.

Musculo-skeletal system

Myalgia Aching muscles; also called fibrositis

Arthralgia Aching joints

Arthritis Swollen, painful joints; not infective, rheumatoid or degenerative arthritis (osteoarthritis)

Central nervous system

Headache Migraine, neuralgia, pins and needles, numbness
Convulsions (*fits*) Allergic in origin when there is no demonstrable cause.
Tinnitus Ringing in the ears
Vertigo Often accompanied by nausea associated with disturbance of the vomiting centre in the brain

Genito-urinary system

Frequent urination, often incorrectly called cystitis; vaginal discharge; some cases of impotence, frigidity and inability to conceive.

Mind and emotions

Behaviour problems 'Dopey' feeling and inability to think clearly; in children, alternating dullness and irritability are common.
Neuroses Especially anxiety neurosis, panic attacks and lack of confidence and energy. Used to be called neurasthenia.
Hypomania and mania; depression Known to psychiatrists as the affective psychoses (affect = mood), these often alternate in the same patient.
Disorders of thought Including delusions and hallucinations (some forms of schizophrenia).

Endocrine system

Hypo- and hyperthyroidism Under- and overactive thyroid gland
Dysmenorrhoea Painful menstruation
Amenorrhoea Failure to menstruate
Menorrhagia Excessively heavy menstruation

At first glance, this list is a formidable hotchpotch of seemingly unrelated conditions, many of which have other well-known causes. Any doctor could be forgiven for accusing me of trying to cram the whole of medicine into my specific adaptive framework. A closer look, however, shows that the net has not been thrown too wide: it includes only the clinical manifestations of allergy (swelling, leakage of fluid and chemical irritation by histamine) as they would affect the three basic tissues of the body: skin and nervous system (ectoderm), muscles, joints and blood vessels (mesoderm) and gut, lungs and mucous membranes (endoderm).

An inherited allergic susceptibility will reveal itself in these basic tissues in one or more of the following ways: where the skin is susceptible we find acne, dandruff, a tendency to develop boils and athlete's foot, eczema, psoriasis, contact dermatitis, drug rashes, heavy body odour and sweating.

Sensitivity of the nervous system may show up as neuritic pain, *tic douloureux*, Bell's palsy, or any one of a whole group of mental and neurological symptoms caused by local swelling and irritation of cells in different parts of the brain. There may also be a general feeling of fatigue, possibly produced by internal swelling of specific cells.

Where the blood vessels are susceptible, we find urticaria, puffiness under the eyes, swollen ankles, alteration in blood pressure, lumbago, sudden redness of one eye and painful periods. Certain types of dizziness may also occur, as in Ménière's disease, resulting from spasm and swelling of blood vessels in the organ of balance and in the area of the brain responsible for the coordination of posture.

Muscle involvement shows itself as cramps and the aches and pains commonly called muscular rheumatism or fibrositis. When the joints are involved, pain and stiffness occur.

A person whose gut and mucous membranes are susceptible may develop styes, mouth ulcers, coated tongue, heavy breath, snoring, sneezing, frequent colds, post-nasal drip, asthma or hay fever. Gastric and duodenal ulcer

83

symptoms, colitis, diarrhoea, constipation, and vaginal discharge also fall into this category, as does the ubiquitous 'cystitis' of women when it is not associated with infection.

Localized allergic reactions should not be seen in isolation, for they penetrate and complicate other medical problems. Abnormal susceptibility to viræ and bacterial infection, for instance, can frequently be ascribed to an allergy that involves the affected tissues, making them more than usually vulnerable to invasion by germs.

The germ theory of disease had an enormous impact on medical science, but we think of germs alone as the enemy. Germs need the right environment in which to grow, and the tissues involved in allergic reactions make ideal seedbeds for bacteria and viruses. Take, for example, the asthmatic, whose illness is – at first, anyway – based entirely on an allergic reaction, a failure to adapt to pollen in the air or to the mites in bedding that have recently been identified as a major cause of allergic asthma. The membranes lining the tubes and air spaces in the asthmatic's lungs become increasingly irritated, providing a perfect breeding ground for the germs that cause bronchitis. Should he be exposed to these germs, chances are the asthmatic will also become a chronic bronchitic before long. If he is a smoker who inhales, the chemical irritants in the tobacco smoke will speed the disease process.

Or take the child with allergic infantile eczema, commonly caused by a failure to adapt to cow's milk. His eczema will gradually become infected through scratching, and he may end up with impetigo, a streptococcal skin infection, in addition to his eczema.

This allergy-based group of common infections includes recurrent styes, sore throats, ear infections and persistent catarrh. (Remember Dr Rinkel's story, pages 58–9). When the specific substances to which the patient is allergic are identified and excluded in such cases, normal resistance to infection is restored and the distressing recurrent bouts of inflammation, previously treated with antibiotics, come to an end. (Remember, too, that allergy to antibiotics can often develop and make matters worse.) This approach, which takes the allergic or adaptive factor into account, enables the doctor to provide his patient with better treatment.

Soon after I learned about food allergy and failure of specific adaptation, I was able, while still a general practitioner, to help clear up for good the constant sore throats, tonsillitis and ear infections that were keeping two children out of school and making their lives a misery. Peter was six and his sister Mary five, and they had both missed so much school that their parents were in despair. One day, on the umpteenth call to one of the children, who was again running a temperature, I sat down with the mother and made a careful inventory of Peter and Mary's diet. The children usually started the day with a bowl of cornflakes, followed by white toast and jam. For lunch they took sandwiches to school – when they were well enough to go – and spent their pocket money on chocolate bars. At mid-morning they drank the one-third of a pint of school milk provided. When they got home about 4 30p.m., their mother had a high tea ready with something cooked: scrambled egg or baked beans on toast, after which they had bread and jam, cake, biscuits and sometimes a banana or orange. Orange or lemon squash was available and at bedtime they had a malted milk drink and an apple.

I explained to the mother, who was a pleasant woman and very fond of her children, that it was quite likely Peter and Mary had become allergic to the items in this diet made from refined starch and sugar, and possibly also to cow's milk and egg. I then designed a menu for them which

85

excluded these things altogether. It went something like this:

Breakfast Grilled bacon, wholemeal fried bread;
or grilled herrings or toasted cheese on wholemeal bread with grilled tomatoes or fresh apple rings.
Mid-morning Go without the school milk, but take home-made lemonade made from fresh lemons and a banana or two.
Lunch Eat the school lunch but not the pudding.
High tea Meat and two vegetables, fresh fruit when in season. Lentils. Nuts of all kinds: brazils, hazel nuts, almonds or peanut butter eaten with a spoon. Fish of all kinds.
Bedtime Hot soup, home-made in a stockpot from the bones and meat left over from the high teas.
No sweets or chocolate of any kind. No squashes or soda-pop.

This was a simple, shot-in-the-dark elimination diet which removed the four most likely food offenders from the children's diet: refined starch (white flour), sugar, cow's milk, and eggs (and chicken, because allergy to chicken often accompanies eggs). I took a calculated risk in allowing cheese, but stipulated that they should not be given it more often than once in three days.

At first it was difficult to persuade the children to stick to this diet, but with a certain amount of bribery in the form of treats and outings and with full cooperation from the school staff, they finally got used to it and even came to prefer it to their old way of eating. The results from the health point of view were most gratifying: fewer colds and sore throats, better school attendance and a pair of much happier children, not to mention parents.

Of course, Peter and Mary still caught the odd cold when colds were going about, but they developed fewer complications and threw them off more easily. Neither child had to have tonsils or adenoids out – an operation which the grandparents had been urging me to arrange.

86

Since these children were too young for food testing and the parents would have found it too difficult, I was limited to trying a modified version of Albert Rowe's procedure. The results were a complete justification of that grand old man's work.

- An approach to illness that considers food and chemical allergy as a factor and failing adaptation to specific substances as a contributory cause, renders a better medical service than the search for a single symptom or complex of symptoms on which the whole illness can be blamed. It is an approach well within the compass of the average general practitioner and a rewarding addition to the kinds of support and treatment he is already able to offer.

Forced to theorize on the basis of incomplete evidence about the causes of their patients' illnesses, doctors on both sides of the Atlantic frequently apply high-sounding descriptive labels to make it seem as if basic disease processes are being named. Since patients are gullible and in no position to argue with the physician, they usually have to accept this kind of 'sucker diagnosis' (as the late Dr Blake Donaldson, New York physician and allergist, used to call it).

In his book *Strong Medicine*[12], Donaldson gives a hair-raising account of one such patient who came to him because she felt 'sick all over', had splitting headaches, colicky abdominal pain and a sense of utter exhaustion. She had been thoroughly gone over by other physicians and surgeons uninterested in allergy. Here are the 'diagnoses' which had been made and for which she had undergone treatment without benefit: duodenal ulcer, low blood pressure, low blood sugar, calcium deficiency, vitamin deficiency, slipped disc (for which she refused an operation), fallen stomach, low thyroid, streptococcus infection, anaemia and high cholesterol.

On a diet of fresh fat meat and water, which completely eliminated the white flour to which Donaldson found her to be sensitive, all her symptoms cleared up within a week or two. Later he was able to expand her diet to include baked potatoes and fresh fruit without bringing her illness back.

chapter five

It will be remembered that Joanna had been admitted for the thirteenth time to Park Prewett after yet another episode of self-injury, accompanied by depressive withdrawal. Six months later she was transferred to the Psychiatric Intensive Care Unit where she was given the benefit of every available treatment, including a high level of nursing and ancillary care, as a last attempt at cure before being considered for a leucotomy. After three weeks in Intensive Care, during which she had not improved, she was shown at the weekly clinical case conference, at which the ten or eleven psychiatrists present agreed that psycho-surgery offered the only hope of remission and that the three children should be taken into care for their own safety. Mine was the only dissenting voice. Her case was so desperate, however, that I was allowed to take her on for food testing even though most of the doctors were highly sceptical of my approach. The mood of the meeting was: 'It is bound to fail, but at least it can do no harm.'

As Joanna had had a full physical examination recently, I did not repeat this, although normally I would give one to a new patient in order to exclude any obvious physical abnormality. Nor did I repeat the routine blood count and biochemical tests which are part of the thorough going-over given all patients taken into Intensive Care. Her tests had all been normal.

She was considerably overweight: 14 stone 1½ pounds at a height of 5 feet 6 inches. She stood or sat about, chain-smoking, looking hunched and dejected, scarcely speaking. She had to be under constant observation because at any moment she might run off, usually into the lavatory, and slash her arms with any cutting object she could get hold of – often a heavy glass ashtray which she smashed on the edge of the WC bowl. The blood and mess of broken glass after these episodes was considerable. Only a couple of weeks before, as duty doctor, I had had to sew up one of these self-inflicted cuts, which was deep and needed three or four sutures. Her forearms were covered with scars. Joanna was always temporarily calmer right after one of these assaults upon herself, which made the task of sewing her up easier and showed that in some way the injury relieved her inner tension, like the man who bangs his head against the wall because he feels so good when he stops.

At 5p.m. on Monday 28 May 1973, I started Joanna on a five-day total fast with nothing but plenty of water to drink. Her drugs were gradually tapered off; this move caused consternation among the staff, who were accustomed to keeping her in what amounted to a chemical strait-jacket. The variety and quantity of medication she was on was prodigious even by psychiatric standards *: 25 mg of imipramine (Tofranil) three times a day, plus 50 mg of trimipramine (Surmontil) at night (these two are powerful anti-depressants), and 5 mg of haloperidol (Serenace) three times a day (haloperidol, a major tranquillizer chemically related to the substance used to knock out wild animals that have to be relocated, is the drug the Russians are said to use on their political/psychiatric

* The names of the drugs in brackets are the trademark names given to them by the drug companies who make them; the other names are the pharmacological names approved by the Ministry of Health.

prisoners). She was also given 100 mg of orphenadrine (Disipal) three times a day to counteract the haloperidol's side-effects – muscular rigidity, tremors and excessive salivation. At night she got 10 mg of nitrazepam (Mogadon), a sleeping pill, and she was down for injections of 10 mg of haloperidol and 10 mg of procyclidine (Kemadrin) as necessary to control her outbursts of slashing and running away. On top of all this, she was getting a tablet of fenfluramine (Ponderax) twice a day for her obesity, and a daily Norinyl contraceptive pill lest she became pregnant – not that she had much sex drive under all this medication and depression, but the policy was 'better safe than sorry'.

During this fast, I took a diet history from Joanna in order to establish exactly what she had been eating and drinking by choice. These diet histories nearly always reveal addiction to certain foods in food-allergy patients like Joanna, and in her case there was obviously addictive drinking of coffee.

Here is a typical day's menu for her:

8.30a.m. Three mugs of instant coffee with milk and plenty of white sugar.

11.00 One or two more similar mugs of coffee.

12.30p.m. (Husband comes home to lunch) Something hot: mince or sausages or eggs and chips or stew (with barley, oxtail, etc). Cheese and biscuits. Glass of orange squash and one or two mugs of coffee.

3.00 More sweet, milky coffee.

6.00 (Family main meal) Scrambled eggs on toast, soup from a can. Bread and butter, cakes and biscuits.

9.00 (TV snack) Sandwiches of cheese or fish paste. Tea with milk and sugar.

Midnight One mug of coffee with milk and sugar as above.
Between-meal snacks if hungry ('fridge raiding'): yogurt or milk.

This is not what dieticians call a balanced diet. Joanna seldom ate fruit or fresh vegetables and she could have done with a decent breakfast, but, as with all food addicts, the abstention from her addictant (sweet coffee) during the hours of sleep stimulated her craving. By morning she was dying for a mug of coffee, which picked her up temporarily and got her going for the day, just as the tobacco addict's first fag in the morning is the only thing that can make him feel 'normal'.

Joanna stuck to her fast and once out of the hangover phase, which lasted two days, she began to look and feel progressively better. The ward staff remarked on the improvement in her appearance, mood and behaviour. Now that she was in a more lucid and cooperative state, I was able to get a more detailed history from her, which strongly confirmed the diagnosis of food and chemical allergy.

For brevity, I will summarize her allergic history in a list of signs and symptoms, in the order in which she gave them to me:

1 Overweight. She had been slim until the age of twenty, after which her weight varied between 9 stone 12 pounds and 15 stone 2 pounds. On the day I saw her, she had lost about half a stone on her total fast and weighed 13 stone 8½ pounds.

2 For years, her nose had itched, her eyes had watered, and she had sneezed repeatedly whenever she put on powder or eye-shadow.

3 Most nights she had bouts of wheezing in bed.

4 She smoked addictively: forty to sixty cigarettes a day.

5 Babycham, a bubbly form of perry, made from pears, made her giddy and happy after four small glasses; this lasted about one hour, after which she would get depressed.

6 She suffered occasionally from palpitations or what doctors call tachycardia: a rapid beating of the heart of which the patient is uncomfortably aware.

7 Occasional constipation.

8 Night cramps.

9 Heavy, drenching sweats (hyperidrosis), not related to exercise.

By 31 May 1973, the third day of her fast, she said she felt much better and 'more in touch', looked more lively, stood up straighter and could smile. The next day she was shown to the weekly ward meeting in the Intensive Care Unit, and managed to sit at the table and give a good account of herself. Previously she either would not attend these meetings or sat slumped and silent until she could get away. The next day, Saturday 2 June, her fast was broken with an individual food ingestion test of braised steak, to which there was no adverse reaction. Thereafter she test-fed four single foods per day, at the ordinary meal times, and nurses recorded her pulse before and after (see Coca's pulse test, page 62).

Green beans and plain boiled rice produced no reaction, but bacon for breakfast on the second day of test-feeding, Sunday 3 June, was followed by a drop in her pulse rate from 100 per minute just before the test feed to 76, ninety minutes later. (A drop of 20 or more is as significant as a rise, and should alert the staff to the possibility that a major reaction is to be expected. In fact she soon went into depression that lasted several hours.)

For supper that same day, after her depression had lifted, we tested eggs – two boiled eggs – and a really severe reaction followed, requiring constant nursing observation and injection of 10 mg of haloperidol to stop her running off and injuring herself. The change in her appearance was striking: she went right back to her hunched, downcast posture and was able to talk about herself only with difficulty and in monosyllables. As she came out of the extreme depression she began to wheeze and described a feeling of constriction in her chest and a sensation of being 'screwed up inside'. By the next morning she was better and the pine-apple juice, turkey and carrots which she had for breakfast, lunch and tea, separately and in that order, had no ill effects. By supper-time, she was normally cheerful and alert. For this test she had tongue, and quickly became tense and agitated and tried to steal food. The agitation soon gave place to depression which lasted until she went to bed feeling very tired.

Testing went on like this for a fortnight, until we had established a fairly wide range of foods which caused no adverse reactions and seven foods which brought her illness back in acute form, within the hour. These were bacon, egg, porridge, veal, tongue, instant coffee and chocolate. On Wednesday 20 June, after she had been on her safe, compatible diet for two days Joanna was again presented at the weekly case conference. She performed very well, chatting happily to everyone, sitting relaxed and attentive, answering the doctors' questions readily and to the point. The medical staff were impressed and urged me to proceed to the next step which was to place in random order five 'safe' and five 'unsafe' foods and give them to Joanna, one per day, down a stomach tube from syringes masked with paper. By this time she had been off all regular medication for two weeks, getting only an occasional injection of haloperidol or diazepam (Valium) to control her in a severe reaction.

At this stage, it may be helpful to look at the pattern of Joanna's reaction to a test feeding with a food to which she has a masked allergy. Definite stages in a reaction were

94

apparent and became recognizable to Joanna herself, as well as the nurses whose job it was to note and evaluate her reactions.

Let us take coffee as an example: for about thirty minutes after drinking it she was stimulated and alert, in high spirits, with a tendency to burst into song and sometimes to dance. This good feeling gradually merged into keyed-up irritability, tension and apprehension. Gradually she became more withdrawn, feeling that she must get away and injure herself. If frustrated in an attempt to slash her arms or escape, she would become tired and depressed, sometimes weeping a little. Mental confusion prevented any real communication at this stage, during which she would usually retire to bed, her limbs and back aching. On waking after an hour or two of sleep she would sometimes have a wheezy chest and would always feel tired and dispirited. Actually slashing her arms would make her feel temporarily better and more relaxed, but the whole cycle would still have to be gone through until she emerged four of five hours later feeling more or less normal, though battered.

The whole reaction from start to finish (i.e. from the time she ate the unsafe food until the reaction abated) would, if untreated, last from six to twenty-four hours, depending on how allergic she was to the particular food, her powers of resistance and general health at the time, and the amount she had eaten. Randolph found that bicarbonate of soda, either taken as a solution in water or injected intravenously, will lessen the signs and symptoms of a reaction, and he has used this method to speed up the work on patients being tested in his surgery in Chicago. I have tried giving patients bicarbonate of soda in these circumstances, but in Joanna's case found it difficult to persuade her to drink it – such was her negativism at these times. Patients who do take it find that it not only relieves their symptoms but also flushes out any offending food that might still be in the intestines, thus helping to cut short the reaction. Why an alkali given in this way should relieve symptoms generally, as well as acting in its time-honoured way as a purgative, is a bit of a mystery. Some years ago an American surgeon, Harry Clark, who was interested in food allergy, suggested an explanation and published it with Randolph in an article entitled 'Sodium bicarbonate in the treatment of allergic conditions'[6]. What they said, in essence, was that in an allergic reaction such as I have described, the local swelling in the target organ tends to reduce the supply of oxygen to the tissues involved and this leads to a local build-up of acid, which can cause the normally alkaline pH of the blood and tissue fluids to shift slightly to the acid side (i.e. towards 7·0 which represents neutrality). This slight shift of pH is what makes the patient feel unwell. Putting in an alkali like bicarbonate of soda, either intravenously or orally, brings the pH back to 7·4 and sets things right. This phenomenon may help to explain the booming sales of commercial antacid, as well as the popularity of cigarette smoking, for cigarette smoke is strongly alkaline and can help to relieve allergic reactions. Doubters can moisten a piece of red litmus paper in distilled water and hold it up in the smoke curling up from a lighted cigarette. The litmus paper will turn blue at once. I once asked a friend who worked in an advertising agency to make me a chart of the sales of cigarettes and antacids since the Second World War: the two lines on the graph went steadily up, year by year, in parallel. All this is speculative, but it is possible that Clark may have been onto something important.

Now to get back to Joanna's case.

Mrs Slade, the hospital dietitian, placed ten foods in

random order: five safe and five unsafe according to the open test feeding just completed. Cod, turkey, cheese, milk and oranges were chosen for the safe foods and coffee, egg, porridge, veal and bacon for the unsafe, or allergenic, ones. They were emulsified with plain water in a blender and drawn up into 50-ml syringes which were covered with opaque paper and marked with a code letter. Only Mrs Slade knew the code.

At 5p.m. on Monday 25 June 1973, the first tube feeding was given. The tube passed easily and there were no adverse reactions afterwards. On breaking the code later, at the end of the tests, this first feeding turned out to be milk – a food to which Joanna had shown no reaction previously. Observations of her reactions were recorded in two ways: by two nurses independently of one another on the form reproduced on page 98, and by Joanna herself on the subjective rating form (page 99), which recorded her own assessment of how she felt before and after the feeding. These forms were prepared specially to cover the particular signs and symptoms Joanna had suffered in the past. The forms were not read immediately, but were put in sealed envelopes for analysis when the syringes were decoded after all the tests had been done.

Joanna was given one tube feeding per day for ten days, always in the afternoon, so that should she have a bad reaction, she would have the whole night to recover. For the rest of the day, at breakfast, lunch and teatime, she was allowed to eat one or two foods per meal, foods to which she had shown no adverse reaction previously. Note that in our hospital all these meals arrive earlier than they would outside: breakfast before 8a.m., lunch at midday and tea at 3p.m.

On the second day of tube feeding, shortly before the test feed was due, Joanna felt hungry and sneaked a bar of

PSYCHIATRIC INTENSIVE CARE UNIT
OBJECTIVE RATING OF REACTIONS TO TEST FEEDINGS

date_____ test code_____

observer_____

0 = none
1 = mild
2 = moderate
3 = severe

	pre-test 10 min	food given	after test 10-min	20 min	1hr	2hr	3hr	4hr
appears anxious								
sweating								
hot and cold flushes								
tremor								
appears depressed								
expresses guilt								
restless								
attempts to run away								
poor concentration								
expressing desire to slash herself								
cheerful								
wheezing								
pulse rate								
any other symptoms								

The form used by Joanna's nurses

PSYCHIATRIC INTENSIVE CARE UNIT
SUBJECTIVE RATING OF REACTIONS TO TEST FEEDINGS

date_____ test code_____ 0 = none
                                                                      1 = mild
observer_____ 2 = moderate
                                                                      3 = severe

	pre-test 10 min	food given	after test 10 min	20 min	1hr	2hr	3hr	4hr
apprehension								
feelings of panic								
sweating								
feels hot or cold								
shivering								
sadness								
guilt								
feeling restless								
desire to run away								
impulse to slash								
headache								
bloated feeling								
tight chest								
difficulty in concentrating								
feeling good								
any other symptoms								

The form used by Joanna
(note that she was not always able to fill this in)

chocolate at about 4p,m. Within five minutes she became excited, and overactive; later she started hitting people indiscriminately, and within an hour began to feel tired and depressed. We omitted the tube feeding that day and let her sleep the reaction off. Next day the tube feeding was moved up to 4p.m. to avoid letting her get too hungry, and there was no more illicit eating.

The testing continued until she had taken all ten foods; then we broke the code and analysed the observation forms. The results – to my relief, because if they had gone wrong I would have looked an awful fool – were entirely consistent with the results obtained by open test feeding. Everyone was delighted. Next day we let Joanna go home, on no drugs and with a menu of safe foods for the next week.

Here are the final results of the tube feeding:

Date fed	Code letter	Food	Reactions (graded 0 to 3)
25.6.73	A	milk	0
26.6.73	sneaked	chocolate	1 to 3
27.6.73	B	orange	0
28.6.73	C	bacon	1 to 3 (particularly bad)
29.6.73	D	cod	0
30.6.73	E	coffee	1 to 3 (bad)
1.7.73	F	egg	1 to 3
2.7.73	G	porridge	1 to 2
3.7.73	H	veal	1 to 3
4.7.73	I	cheese	0 to 2 (thought to be an extension of the cumulative reaction to previous four bad foods, which happened to come in succession).

Finally, on 5 July, when she was feeling fine, we did a tube test with plain distilled water to see if there would be any 'psychological' or suggestive effect. The reaction was entirely negative.

The menu I gave Joanna to take home was varied and somewhat flexible, in that I allowed between-meal snacks of specified foods and gave her alternative choices if an item on the menu happened to be unavailable or too expensive. The plan was for her to work through the whole menu in a week and then go back to the beginning and start again. If she broke the diet and ate a forbidden item (a list of forbidden foods was given to her, to her husband and to her general practitioner, who by this time was well in the picture), she was to take nothing but plain water until she felt normal again.

A person with an allergic constitution or inheritance can create new allergies by eating the same compatible food too often. So in the rotating compatible diet I made up for Joanna, I attempted to vary the foods from day to day so that she would not eat the same thing too often. Many people follow a very monotonous, repetitive menu out of habit, and thus run the risk of creating food allergies in themselves. It will be seen that Joanna's diet was not unduly dull or restrictive.

The cost of some of the items in this menu proved a problem, but Joanna and her husband showed considerable ingenuity in finding and test-feeding cheaper substitutes. At first I called regularly at the house to go over the menu with them and advise on any difficulties that arose.

Joanna found a job almost at once and has kept it ever since apart from two short breaks when she had to be readmitted to hospital for stabilization after breaking her diet. Her GP has gradually taken over her management,

	Breakfast	Lunch	Tea	Supper	Snacks
Monday	orange juice (fresh)	lamb chops and peas	black tea	beef mince, hamburgers and tomatoes	banana
Tuesday	toast and butter	chicken, green beans	glass of milk	corn on the cob	sardines
Wednesday	pineapple juice	beef sausages, butter beans	half-pint Guinness	avocado with oil and vinegar	Cheddar cheese
Thursday	half a grapefruit	lamb, French beans	half-pint cider	pilchards	pears
Friday	lemon juice and water	cold lamb, green peppers	Bovril	Welsh rarebit	peaches
Saturday	toast and butter	roast turkey and potato	milk	rabbit and peas	apples
Sunday	cornflakes milk	cold turkey, lettuce	light ale	poached fish	Cheshire cheese

For substitution, any of these:
celery, Brussels sprouts, parsnips, chicory, cherries, strawberries, raspberries, spinach, hare, venison, tripe, shrimps, cod's roe, rice
Forbidden foods, not to be eaten in any circumstances:
Pork in any form (bacon, ham, sausages), egg, porridge (or anything made of oats), veal, tongue, coffee, chocolate. (Later tea was added to this list because it began to upset her)

and after she had been home three months, sent me the report on her quoted on page 24.

The fact that allergy to certain foods has been shown to give rise to certain behaviour patterns in a patient like Joanna does not mean that she may not also have an attention-seeking streak in her personality. Such a person may be expected to use her knowledge of the bad effects of certain foods upon herself to gain unconsciously desired ends, particularly when frustrated or angry with others in the ordinary course of living. Psychotherapy can help overcome this.

chapter six

The most commonly asked question about food allergy and specific adaptation is 'How can people be allergic to ordinary foods like bread and potatoes which they like and eat every day without trouble?'

In ordinary food allergy the allergic person knows what affects him badly, avoids it if possible and is incapacitated immediately if he accidentally eats it. In masked food allergy on the other hand, the victim feels better after a meal containing his allergen, provided he eats the offending food often – at least once a day and preferably at every meal. The hangover which develops when the regular dose of a specifically sensitizing food or chemical is missed will last from one to three days, gradually lessening in severity until the victim emerges feeling well. At any time during that period, the victim can terminate the hangover by taking another dose of the allergen, and most people with this illness learn to keep a supply on hand – chocolate on the bedside table, for instance, or an emergency store of cigarettes. We all know cigarette addicts who give up smoking for a day or two and feel so awful that they have to start again. The blessed relief of tension and malaise following the first drag is wonderful to behold and certainly has more to do with allergy than with alkali in the smoke.

Masking in food allergy means reduction or abolition of allergic symptoms – headache, depression, catarrh, whatever they may be – by eating a specific food within the period of time (up to three days) in which a person is reacting to a previous feeding of that food to which he has a masked allergy. A reaction in this case means an altered response, a response not experienced by non-allergic people; it has two phases – a pick-up or lift, followed by a hangover – the whole process taking up to three days. The symptoms in the hangover when a person is in the adapting stage two (or stage of resistance) are the same as the symptoms which come on immediately on exposure when a person is in stage one (alarm) or in stage three (exhaustion). In stage two, however, repeated exposures mask the hangover symptoms by keeping one picked-up.

Many years ago, before I cut eggs out of my diet, I had, like Dr Rinkel, a masked allergy to them. I used to eat them often and I noticed, when I was a student and doing my own cooking, that I could work particularly well after I had eaten an omelet. Next morning, after an evening at the textbooks, I would wake depressed, with a headache which lasted until I had eaten two boiled eggs for breakfast. Then I felt fine until the afternoon, when, unless I had eaten eggs for lunch, I would fall asleep during lectures. None of this meant anything significant to me while it was happening. Allergy to eggs was the last thing I suspected. I tried to prevent sleeping during lectures by drinking strong coffee after lunch, which I found only partially successful. I now find myself allergic to coffee, so I avoid it also. These are the effects of food allergy as it most commonly exists, and they are the reverse of the popular conception of allergic reactions. Instead of feeling bad at once, the patient feels better and naturally thinks the food agrees with him. Unpleasant symptoms connected with masked allergy only appear later, if more of the food is not eaten, and the hangover stage is entered.

Some years ago, a psychiatrist friend of mine heard me

lecture on the subject and realized that he must have a masked allergy to bacon, which he liked very much and always ate for breakfast. For some time, my friend had noticed that he got more and more tired during his afternoon clinics. His fatigue became so disabling that he had to cancel some of his appointments and go to sleep on the couch in his own consulting room. After hearing me talk about masked allergy he told me about his sleepiness and I suggested that he omit bacon and all pork products from his diet. The sequel was quite funny.

Very soon after stopping eating bacon and pork, his former energy and zest for work returned. He was so pleased that he told his colleagues about what had happened. They laughed and said that he was romancing, but just to be sure they decided to test the idea. One of the doctors persuaded the cook in the hospital to slip some chopped bacon into a steak pie which was served to my friend for lunch. After only a few mouthfuls he fell fast asleep at the table like the dormouse at the Mad Hatter's teaparty. The doctors who were in on the experiment were impressed and some of them even admitted that there might be something to masked food allergy after all.

Masking is characteristic of stage two of the specific adaptation syndrome, when the subject is adapting well and his defensive glands and their hormones are in good working order. But, as in Selye's general adaptation syndrome (see page 51), the stages of specific adaptation are a continuum, ending in stage three, towards which the victim is moving inexorably. As stage three is entered, there is exhaustion of the hormonal and enzyme resources needed to remain normal in the face of the stress exerted by a particular allergenic food. Now every meal brings not a temporary pick-up but a devastating onset of symptoms. A diagram showing Selye's three stages of adaptation to a stressor (in this case an allergenic food) will help to make this clear:

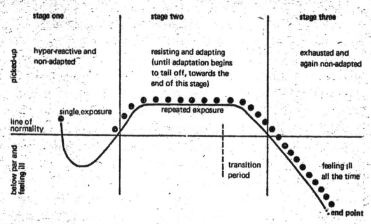

In the transition period between stages two and three ever more frequent and larger doses are needed to produce the same level of alertness which passes more and more rapidly into deeper and more lingering hangover symptoms, so that the victim comes to spend a greater part of each day feeling rotten. This can be shown in the following diagram, which I owe to Dr Randolph:

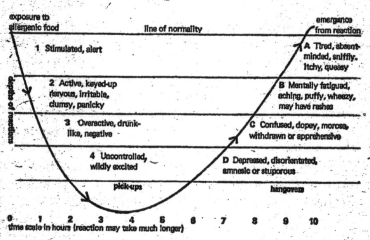

The ten-hour time scale shown here is arbitrary, as the duration of reaction varies from person to person and from food to food. As a general rule, it may be said that three days is the longest a reaction will last, and that, as adaptation fails, the pick-ups grow shorter and the hangovers longer. This is to be expected if Selye and Randolph are right in supposing that the alert state results from the release of stimulating, adaptive adrenal hormones. As fatigue or the wearing out of the adrenal responses makes these hormones less available, hangovers begin to predominate. It is significant, in this connection, that children and adolescents afflicted with specific adaptive illness show mainly the overactive, stimulated side of the reaction – presumably because their hormonal adaptive responses are more vigorous than those of older people, in whom the picture of failing adaptation is more depressive, dopey and withdrawn. Early in the illness, pick-ups may go only to level 2 before moving across into level B on the hangover side. Later, as adaptation fails, pick-ups may go to levels 3 or 4 and the victim may experience really severe hangover symptoms in the corresponding levels C and D.

Before she was treated by elimination dieting, Joanna had come to exist mainly at level 2B (see diagram), occasionally dipping into 3C and 4D, at which times hospitalization and massive sedation were required. Because she was so allergic to coffee and drank it so often and in such large quantities, her adaptive resources were kept at full stretch, taking her from keyed-up nervousness, irritability and panic (eased by slashing) through suicidal depression, dopey confusion, wheezing and brain fatigue, and back again to panic and nervousness. Even during the early years of her illness, she rarely came out of a reaction feeling normal.

When a victim is young, in the early stages of this illness and adapting fairly well, the alert state can be maintained during the day by regular mealtime consumption of the allergen at four-hourly intervals. Hangover symptoms will come on only in the early hours of the morning when the masking effect has had time to wear off. The victim will wake at around 5a.m. with a headache, feeling depressed. A bedside snack of the food involved is more effective than a sleeping pill against this type of insomnia.

Here's a case that illustrates the drift into the hangover zone and the deepening of the reactions in a person heavily and regularly exposed to allergens.

The patient, a pleasant, unmarried woman of thirty-six, first came to my surgery to ask for a prescription for eight bottles of a nasal decongestant. She said she had developed a blocked nose five years earlier, and now she needed eight bottles every two weeks to shrink her mucous membranes and keep her nasal passages clear.

I supplied her with this medicine for some time, then suggested she should be skin tested for allergens to see if we could not desensitize her.

Skin tests showed she was highly allergic to dusts and moulds, but before I could give her more than the first few desensitizing injections she moved back to her home town in the North, where from some reason she failed to complete the course of injections.

When she returned to my neighbourhood two years later, she came to me again, saying that now her nasal symptoms were much less troublesome, but she had begun to suffer from lack of confidence, inability to concentrate, and sudden attacks of irrational panic.

She sent for me or my assistant urgently on several occasions because of acute panic and inability to leave the house. My colleague was convinced she was suffering from hysteria.

In my opinion, she was not hysterical but a most intelligent and cooperative patient suffering from masked allergy. I persuaded her to let me determine what her allergies were by a modification of Rinkel's and Randolph's methods. Let us recall the levels of specific allergic reaction during failing adaptation

Level of normality

	A absent-minded, tired, sniffly, itchy, queasy
depths of hangover	**B** mentally fatigued, achy, puffy, wheezy, may have rashes
	C confused, dopey, morose, withdrawn or panicky
	D depressed, disorientated, amnesic or stuporose

I judged my patient to have been living at level A most of the time when I first saw her, and now to be at C. She was approaching stage three, her specific adaptive energy almost exhausted.

The major offenders turned out to be wheat, Indian tea, house dust and moulds. Elimination of Indian tea and all cereal foods quickly brought her up to level A. Confusion and panic disappeared, and she was able to go back to work, though handicapped by a return of her nasal congestion.

A full course of hyposensitization with mould and dust vaccine cleared her nose and she is now well.

During her individual food ingestion tests, after a five-day fast had brought her back to the hyper-reactive, non-adapted state of stage one, single feedings of white bread and Indian tea brought on her old symptoms in acute, easily recognizable form. She was able to observe herself going quickly through the stages of her illness: stimulation, anxiety, agitation and panic, moving over into depression and dopeyness, and finally emerging via mental fatigue and lack of confidence to the nasal stuffiness for which she had first consulted me. This had never left her, because it was due to dusts and moulds, not food allergy.

Food sensitivity usually goes along with specific sensitivity to other allergens like house dust, moulds, pollens, tobacco, paint and hydrocarbon emissions. The clinical effects of these sensitivities overlap and reinforce each other. A patient of mine who is very sensitive to the fumes of indoor gas heaters and is also addicted to cigarettes, finds that she is driven to smoke more if she has had to spend time in a shop heated by unvented gas. At such times she also craves alcohol.

A pertinent question at this stage is: what drives the allergic person who is adapting to specific substances to go after these substances in a compulsive way? Is he not simply weak-willed? Having talked to many of these patients and having suffered from specific adaptive illness myself, I know that this is not so. Specific allergic adaptation to foods and chemicals is an addiction as devastating as addiction to tobacco or drugs. In my opinion, only heroin or morphine addiction are more potent and destructive than severe food addiction, which I would put on a par with alcoholism.

An allergic patient experiencing a reaction feels very much below par and may have symptoms like mental fatigue and inability to think clearly, which seriously interfere with performance and judgement. A disabling bone-tiredness is also common. The victim may suffer various local allergic symptoms as well, such as skin irritation, abdominal pains and headache. The symptoms are generally accompanied by a strong craving for something to eat, drink or smoke which will put an end to the baffling sense of inner tension and unease.

All this may sound quite artificial and unreal to a non-allergic person. To anyone who has experienced this illness, however, it will be all too familiar.

part three

chapter seven

Over the last seventeen years, during the time that I have been interested in the field of clinical ecology, I have met many doctors whose work confirms much of what I have written in this book.

I became involved in clinical ecology via an interest in obesity so I will mention first those doctors who treated fat patients with a Stone-Age-type, pre-cereal diet (like the one advocated by me in *Eat Fat and Grow Slim*[22]). All of them found, as I had, that the avoidance of starches and sugars cured not only corpulence but also a wide variety of chronic ailments without apparent connection with obesity. I classify these four doctors, whom I met in America and Canada in 1958, as anti-cereal doctors using a simple form of elimination dieting.

Dr Ray Lawson was a surgeon at one of the biggest hospitals in Montreal and surgical consultant to the Canadian Arctic Medical Service. Some of his Eskimo patients in the far north were still eating their old high-fat, high-protein, non-cereal diet, which seemed to him to keep them remarkably fit and give them great powers of endurance. He decided to try to lose some unnecessary weight by following an Eskimo diet himself, an enterprise in which he was completely successful. Just before I visited him, he had confounded his personal physician by curing himself of an attack of jaundice. His doctor had been treating him with orthodox methods, including a low-fat diet, without much success. Dr Lawson switched to large doses of double cream, and promptly got well. An article about him and his high-fat eating was published in the popular Canadian magazine *Maclean's*, and caused quite a stir.

After seeing Dr Lawson I visited the late Dr Alfred Pennington of New Jersey, who was consultant physician to Du Pont, the vast chemical company. Soon after he joined Du Pont, he was asked to develop a reducing plan for the company's overweight executives. He told me that most of them had high blood pressure and were potential stroke- and heart-attack victims.

After going through the literature on obesity and working with Dr Blake Donaldson, Pennington came to the conclusion that obesity in some people is caused by an inability to use carbohydrates for anything except making surplus fat. He suggested that there might be a block on the metabolic pathway which prevented sugars, once absorbed, from being released as energy in the body, and he postulated a short cut into the fat stores with subsequent difficulty in getting the fat out again for conversion into energy.

This theory came in for a good deal of criticism from physiologists and other experts, but no one could deny the success of the slimming programme Pennington designed for his fat executives. In fact the women's magazines took up his diet in a big way – rather to his annoyance, as he was a quiet, scientific man who valued his professional privacy.

The diet he prescribed completely eliminated foods of cereal origin, i.e. everything containing starches or sugars; it was virtually an all-meat diet with the fat left in. When I lunched with him at his house I found he practised what he preached: we had an all-meat meal. He told me that he gave the Du Pont executives about 3000 calories a day in the form of fat meat and that on this regime they lost at the rate of two to three pounds per week. They liked the diet, and by the time their weight had returned to normal, their blood pressure had come down to normal too.

The relationship between obesity and high blood pressure is recognized by doctors all over the world, and the type of high blood pressure known as 'idiopathic' (of unknown cause) is one of the commonest stress disorders of twentieth-century civilized countries, crippling millions every year. It is a forerunner of strokes and coronary thrombosis. I believe that it and its associated obesity are both diseases of maladaptation to certain foods and chemicals we have been eating in increasing quantities over the past sixty to seventy years.

From Pennington I went on to Minneapolis to talk to Dr George L. Thorpe, a general practitioner from Wichita in Kansas, who was attending the 1958 annual meeting of the American Medical Association. At the previous annual meeting in New York in 1957, Thorpe had been chairman of the Section of General Practice and had made the cereal-elimination approach to overweight the subject of his address.

Thorpe told me that he hated to call his method a diet. 'Proper eating is the normal and complete answer to the problem of excess weight,' he said. 'The words diet and dieting should be avoided.

'Several years ago,' Thorpe went on, 'while I was considering a personal problem of excess weight, it became evident that huge numbers of calories in my daily total came from three to four large glasses of milk, two to three bottles of soft drinks, numerous slices of bread, and an educated taste for cookies, candy and sweets in general, all of which are concentrated carbohydrates. Cereal grains, historically, were cultivated in order that limited agriculture areas might supply food to support population densities not otherwise possible. They are concentrated forms of food, readily assimilated by the body, containing small residue of bulk, and so may be eaten in quantities far in excess of the calorie needs, without sensation of fullness. All carbohydrate foods and most drinks fall into this category, either by virtue of their origin or the reaction of the body to them. Milk is actually a liquid infantile food, the use of which man has carried over into his adult life and which, in general, satisfies the definition of concentrated carbohydrate.

'The simplest to prepare and most easily obtainable high-protein, high-fat, low-carbohydrate diet and the one that will produce the most rapid loss of weight without hunger, weakness, lethargy or constipation is made up of meat, fat and water. The total quantity eaten is not important, but the ratio of three parts of lean to one part fat must be maintained, as any decrease in the fat portion will reduce the weight loss.

'Black coffee, clear tea and water are used without restriction. Reduction of salt, while not required, will increase the speed of weight loss.'

The last doctor I met was the late Blake Donaldson (he died in 1963). When I saw him at his clinic in New York I found that not only was he slimming fat patients on a cereal-elimination diet, but he was using this diet and a graduated system of simple exercises to clear up a whole variety of chronic disorders in a most remarkable manner. I saw elderly rheumatic patients made supple and pain-free, martyrs to migraine relieved of their headaches and asthmatics helped to breathe freely again. In an interview in 1962, when he came to London to visit a patient, Donaldson told me how he did it.

DR MACKARNESS When and how did you first come on the ideas which led you to write your book *Strong Medicine*[12]?
DR DONALDSON About 1919. I was faced with the problem

120

of people with heart disease, fat people who were short of breath, had swollen feet (oedema) and could not lose weight. I tried them for a year on a low-calorie diet, with a very bad result. At the end of the year practically none had lost weight, they were still breathless and had not lost their oedema.

I decided to try something new. I went to the American Museum of Natural History and consulted the curator there and asked him what the teeth of the people were like in the old days – because, as you know, all the cells in the body have common qualities, then specialize afterwards. If you can find the best food for teeth, to prevent holes in the teeth, you have perhaps got the best foods for stomachs and hearts and everything else. So I wanted to see what teeth were like in the dawn of history. They showed me skulls from the old Eskimo burial grounds; people who lived on nothing but caribou meat and walrus – essentially fat meat – and they had astonishingly good teeth.

It occurred to me that it might be the primitive nature of the food that prevented dental caries, and I came away from there determined to try primitive foods as a basis for any sensible way of taking weight off fat people with heart disease.

DR M. How long was it after getting this idea that you made it routine and based your whole practice on it?

DR D. Well, of course, in those days we were very much frightened that if you ate meat alone you would get something called acidosis [now called ketosis]; that the meat was just too acid and needed starch to neutralize the acid.

With a good deal of fear and trembling I gave these fat cardiacs nothing whatever but fresh meat, without salt, and potato in deference to the idea that you would get acidosis if you did not have some starch, and black coffee.

I found that many of them lost weight beautifully at the

rate of seven pounds per month. But there were others who did not lose. So again – with considerable fear and trepidation – we tried cutting out the potato, and just gave them meat and coffee. And apparently we struck something that was of great practical value. We found out the patients could live on just fresh meat and a cup of coffee three times a day, and lose weight at the rate of three pounds a week. (You don't want to lose weight much faster than that, otherwise the skin becomes wrinkled.)

Now we are fairly convinced that flour is the root of all evil. It's too concentrated a food.

Mind you, when you make such an arbitrary remark as that, you should remember that there are twenty per cent of people who can eat and drink anything and maintain a normal weight, feel fine, reproduce and live a normal span of years. But it is the other eighty per cent in which we are interested. There are a great many of us who get overweight or develop many unpleasant allergic symptoms when we eat flour.

DR M. After they've improved and lost their excess weight have you tried reintroducing flour to these patients on a test basis to see whether their obesity comes back?

DR D. Yes. And every time I've failed to show that they can tolerate it. The moment flour is introduced, their weight goes right up again.

When you reduce their weight to normal you have to prove their weight can stay normal; that's very important. You have to get them thin enough so that they can eat four things with a meal and show no gain in weight. They have to be able to eat fat meat with salt, potato with butter, raw fruit and a full cup of coffee three times a day and show no gain in weight.

DR M. And they may have unlimited quantities. There is no restriction on the amount?

DR D. No, there is no restriction on the amount.

DR M. How many patients over the last forty years have you treated on this basis?

DR D. About seventeen thousand. I now have a group of about fifteen hundred patients over the age of seventy, who have avoided flour for between five and forty years and have kept primitive food as their basic way of maintaining health.

DR M. This is what I call a Stone-Age diet. Would you agree with that description? It is a pre-cereal diet.

DR D. Well, I should say that it is perhaps six thousand years old and twenty years ahead of its time. I think this will be a popular idea in twenty years, that flour is a bad thing for about eighty per cent of the population.

DR M. And do you also ban all carbohydrate derivatives – sugar, chocolate, etc?

DR D. Once you have an allergic fat person under control you reduce that person's weight to normal. I find that I am unable to feed them sugar in any form, and unable to feed them flour, without bringing back their obesity and their allergic symptoms.

Support for the idea that certain foods and food additives can cause serious mental illness in some susceptible people has come from recent dietary experiments in schizophrenia.

The word schizophrenia, meaning literally 'split mind', was first used by the German-Swiss psychiatrist Eugen Bleuler in 1911 as a better term for the mental disease known until then as *dementia praecox* (premature loss of mental function). Its cause is still unknown and it is a most tragic illness because it affects mainly young people, starting in the late teens and early twenties. Schizophrenia is a psychotic illness, a form of insanity in which the victim loses touch with reality and is afflicted by bizarre oddities of thought, feeling and behaviour. There is incongruity between thought and feeling – a patient will laugh while telling you of some horrible pain he is suffering – and there are delusions, held with the utmost conviction, and hallucinations. Schizophrenics may have tactile hallucinations, but more often they hear voices. In a ward full of schizophrenics, you will see some of them answering their hallucinatory voices.

The first paper I saw written by a psychiatrist on dietary factors in schizophrenia appeared in 1969. It was by F. Curtis Dohan, a doctor at the hospital of the University of Pennsylvania in Philadelphia.[11]

The world-wide incidence of schizophrenia is remarkably constant most of the time. Between 0·85 and 1·2 per cent of the population is affected; it is by no means a rare disease. Dohan pointed out, however, that the incidence of schizophrenia had dropped in occupied countries during the Second World War, but had risen to the normal level soon afterwards, when food became more plentiful. Wondering whether restriction of cereals during the War had anything to do with it, Dohan devised a test: he divided one of his schizophrenic wards into two groups, restricting cereals in one group, and giving the ordinary hospital diet, rich in starch, to the other. Drugs were withheld from both groups so as not to obscure the issue. Before long, a change in the behaviour of one group became apparent: the patients on the no-cereal diet were more approachable, their thoughts were less disordered, and some who had never left the ward were able to go out to work or to go home. The other group remained as deluded and hallucinated and psychotic as ever.

Dohan concluded that the basis of the illness in some schizophrenics was a biochemical abnormality which upset their brain chemistry whenever substances present in wheat got into the bloodstream.

Dohan soon linked his work on schizophrenia to parallel studies of another illness much more firmly associated with wheat intolerance: coeliac disease, a wasting disease of children characterized by abdominal distension, pain, and diarrhoea with the passage of large quantities of fat. The word coeliac means 'related to the belly' and the documented history of the illness goes back to 1888 when Dr Samuel Gee of St Bartholomew's Hospital in London first described it. Its cause remained a mystery for many years, until several paediatricians during the Second World War tried treating coeliacs by elimination of all cereal grains, a method that brought some gratifying results. The reason for the success of the cereal restriction was discovered in 1950 by a Dutch doctor, W. K. Dicke, who wrote his doctoral thesis on coeliac disease.[8, 9] He was able to show that the factor in wheat and rye which harmed the coeliac children was not the starch, but a part of the protein called gluten. Other investigators showed that substances related to gluten in oats and barley could also cause coeliac disease. Thus was born the gluten-free diet which today is followed by all diagnosed coeliacs. And it keeps them well.

The evidence which led Dohan to postulate a link between coeliac disease and schizophrenia was as follows[10]:

1 Adult schizophrenics show a higher-than-chance incidence of coeliac disease in childhood.

2 Adult coeliacs show a higher-than-average incidence of severe mental illness.

3 In both child and adult coeliacs, behaviour disturbances can be produced by introducing gluten into their diet, and can be relieved by a gluten-free diet.

4 In patients with both coeliac disease and schizophrenia, an intensification of the symptoms of one disease is accompanied by an intensification of the symptoms of the other disease.
5 The tendency to develop both diseases is inherited, i.e. it runs in families.

Dohan tested out his hypotheses by putting patients with a first attack of schizophrenia on a gluten-free diet and comparing them with patients taking foods that contained gluten. Those on the gluten-free diet did much better.

For my final confirmatory evidence, I would like to return to ulcerative colitis, which I mentioned on page 57. In this case, the food allergen was cow's milk, another relatively new food to a species like man who lived for millions of years on a diet of fat meat and water.

Because people began drinking cow's milk before they learned to bake bread, allergy or intolerance to cow's milk is an older phenomenon than allergy to wheat. This probably explains why cow's milk allergy is more widely recognized and has been more carefully studied than allergy to foods of cereal origin. Even so, it is only since 1960 that more than a handful of doctors have begun to appreciate the full extent of the damage done by milk to those unfortunate people who cannot take this supposedly most innocuous of all foods.

Any future medical historian of the mid-twentieth century is bound to be critical of the way doctors have ignored the published evidence incriminating cow's milk as one of the causes of ulcerative colitis, a disabling and sometimes fatal disease whose victims are often young adults. Many doctors feel that the only way to treat ulcerative colitis is to perform a colostomy or an ileostomy, both mutilating operations that can be psychologically devastating to the victim.

In January 1961, Professor S. C. Truelove, head of the Nuffield Department of Clinical Medicine at Oxford, published the results of several years' work with ulcerative colitis patients in his wards at the Radcliffe Infirmary[37]. His opening paragraph summed up the medical world's confusion in relation to this disease.

'The aetiology of ulcerative colitis remains obscure. Infective, allergic, nutritional and psychosomatic theories have been advanced, but there is no general agreement that any one of these is an adequate explanation. One result is that medical treatment has been forced to develop on the basis of trial and error. The lack of universal efficacy of our present medical measures is apparent from the fact that total colectomy [surgical removal of the colon] is necessary in some patients. The need to find specific factors in the causation of the disease is obvious.'

He went on to describe the work he had done with his ulcerative colitis patients.

'During the last few years a group of patients with ulcerative colitis has been recognized, in whom removal of milk (and protein milk-products such as cheese) from the diet has been followed by marked improvement in the clinical course of the disease. In several of these patients milk has been reintroduced into the diet, and in every instance this has been followed by a frank attack of ulcerative colitis. The object of the present article is to describe these observations and to discuss their implications.

'There is nothing new in the idea that particular foods may play a part in the aetiology of ulcerative colitis. Andresen (1942)[2] considered that ulcerative colitis was often due to food allergy, giving the figure of "at least 66 per cent of cases". Among the items of food which he considered had been responsible among his patients, milk was outstanding, being incriminated as one factor in 84 per cent of the patients whom he judged to be suffering from food allergy, and being, in his opinion, the sole factor in 40 per cent of them. Other offending items of food were eggs, wheat, potatoes, oranges and tomatoes. He advised the use of special allergy-test diets in order to detect the harmful items of food.

'Likewise, Rowe (1944)[32] considered that ulcerative colitis might be caused by severe allergic reactivity in the colonic mucosa, similar to that which in the skin is responsible for atopic dermatitis. He found that skin tests were useless and recommended elimination diets not greatly dissimilar to those used by Andresen. He obtained remissions in ten out of fourteen patients by these diets.'

I have dwelt rather extensively on ulcerative colitis, because it is a disease which illustrates very well one of the main points of this book: that illnesses which many doctors today regard as psychosomatic (caused by the mind influencing the body), and try – unsuccessfully – to treat on psychotherapeutic lines are really somatopsychic (caused by the body influencing the mind and behaviour).

There is no suggestion that Rowe, Andresen or Truelove, who have between them seen a great many cases, regard ulcerative colitis as psychologically determined. Is it not reasonable to suppose that a person suffering from agonizing abdominal pains and intermittent bloody diarrhoea at all times of the day and night might become mentally upset, worried and even aggressive towards doctors who persistently suggest that the condition is all in the mind?

chapter eight

Many people, when they first learn of the dietary approach to physical and mental illness, want to try it out on themselves immediately and to these people I want to give a word of warning.

Medicine and psychiatry are vast subjects, and doctors bring to their practice a background of accumulated knowledge and experience which it has taken them years to acquire. Before you even consider testing yourself for masked allergy as a cause of whatever ails you, *please* consult with your general practitioner and undergo whatever tests or examinations by specialists he advises.

Only after you have been told by both your GP and a specialist that they can find no cause for your trouble should you start to carry out – with your GP's approval and cooperation – the tests and procedures described in this book and now summarized in this chapter.

Let us assume that you have had all the necessary consultations and tests and remain a patient with a chronic illness of indeterminate origin and diagnosis. You have lots of failed treatments behind you, and you still feel sick in one part of your body or mind, or just sick all over. There are as yet no clinical ecology units in England where you can be admitted for working out your possible allergies. My own special three-bed unit, which I was promised, has not yet materialized because of shortage of NHS money; I have only an out-patient clinic. So you have to undergo the investigations and testing either at home with the help of your GP, or at a hospital out-patient department or allergy clinic with a specialist who is prepared to work with you.

If you are as ill as Joanna was, it would be very difficult to carry out the procedures described in Chapter 5 anywhere but in a psychiatric hospital. Joanna's reactions to some of her food tests were so violent that skilled staff and emergency drugs were necessary to prevent her from injuring herself. But for those whose symptoms are less severe, though still troublesome and disabling, here is a programme that I have been sending out in letter form to interested patients referred to me by their doctors.

Food allergy in relation to the treatment of certain cases of mental and physical disorder

I assume that your GP and the hospital to which he may have referred you have ruled out the possibility of other serious physical or mental illness, and I hope that now your GP thinks it worth while, in view of your long and unresolved illness, to assist you in determining whether food allergy is a possible cause of your trouble. In return for a little of his time initially, he will gain a happier, healthier patient who will need comparatively little of his time in the future. Perhaps you would like to show him this letter.

Briefly, the method is as follows:

1 Five days' total fast on spring water only. (The idea is to avoid chlorine and other contaminants. Bottled Malvern water or distilled water will do.) Drugs should be tapered off.

2 If you are feeling considerably better by the end of the five-day fast, then masked or hidden allergy to foods or their chemical additives must be suspected. If you do not improve, then food allergy is *not* a cause.

3 During the fast, make a list of *all* foods and drinks you consume more often than once every three days. Those you take daily or more often, and like well, are to be particularly suspected.

4 After the five-day fast, each evening, instead of your normal evening meal, have a large helping of one of the suspected foods or beverages, and *take it by itself*, with nothing but water to drink if you are thirsty. If, within an hour or two, your symptoms come back, then that food must go on your blacklist and must be avoided in the future. (Omit breakfast and lunch at first until you have some proved-safe foods.)

A bad reaction may be terminated by taking the following: mix 1 part potassium bicarbonate with 2 parts sodium bicarbonate, and take a tablespoonful in a half-pint of warm water, well stirred. These alkaline salts can be obtained quite cheaply without prescription from your chemist. Besides being laxative and emptying the bowel rapidly of food residue, they have antidote properties because of their alkalinity.

Fast again until all symptoms have gone, then do another test. It is best to carry out one test per day and to do it in the evening. That way, should you have a bad reaction, you will have the whole night in which to recover.

This type of one-food-per-day testing can, obviously, best be tolerated by overweight people. If you are already too thin when you start, you may experience great hunger. To relieve hunger pangs, fill up between tests with helpings of single foods that you never normally eat and that are unrelated to the foods you have been eating often. This may mean choosing some fairly exotic things such as venison, fresh salmon or trout, avocadoes, rabbit or pheasant. Choose meats and unusual vegetables if possible, because allergies to these foods are not common. Later, as your food testing progresses, you can fill up with foods that have been proved through testing to be safe for you.

No food can be considered safe unless you have tested it after five days of strict avoidance and are feeling well at the time of the test. If it does not make you feel ill under these conditions, then you can go on eating it.

5 When you have finished your testing, make a list of foods to which you have shown no reaction. Those are the only foods you

should eat. When in doubt about any food, leave it out of your diet for five days and test it on the sixth day.

6 If you suspect food additives rather than the food itself, first test a pure version of the food, grown organically and prepared without commercial contaminants. For example, if bread is in question, first try eating bread made from compost-grown whole-wheat flour. If that does not affect you badly, test a commercial white loaf. If only the commercial white flour is bad for you, stick to products made only from compost-grown whole wheat. The same principle applies to other foods, including fruits, vegetables and meats.

7 While doing your food testing, keep a food diary, listing everything you eat and drink and the time at which you take it. On the facing page describe how you feel after eating the food, and list any symptoms. A pattern may emerge that will be of interest to you and your doctor.

Several books have been published on this subject, but they are all rather difficult to get hold of. They are: Arthur F. Coca, *Familial Nonreaginic Food-Allergy*[7]; Albert H. Rowe, *Clinical Allergy*[31]; Blake Donaldson, *Strong Medicine*[12] and T. G. Randolph, *Human Ecology and Susceptibility to the Chemical Environment*[27].

Another word of warning: there is an addictive element in food allergy, and you may well get a 'hangover' during the first day or two of your fast. But persevere and do not cheat. In addition, when you are reacting to a food you may crave to eat more of it, or to consume other things to which you may also be sensitive, like alcoholic drinks and sweets. Willpower is needed.

The method of uncovering masked allergies to foods and chemicals outlined above is based on fasting to take you from adapted stage two to non-adapted stage one, when a test feeding will unmask the allergy by causing an immediate reaction. The disadvantage of this method, which involves eating a substantial portion of the suspect food, is that it is slow: adverse reactions take a long time – up to three days – to clear up, and you must feel completely well before you try another test. To avoid this difficulty, I have been using the Provocative Sublingual Drop Test at my hospital, sometimes with groups of five or six patients at one time. This method will appeal to people who know other sufferers and can join together to form a group.

The drop test itself is very simple. The patient makes a list of the foods he or she likes and eats often. (In order to be valid, the test must be preceded by five days' avoidance of these foods.) Uncontaminated small samples of each of these foods are collected in clean china cups or glasses. Each sample is dropped into an electric blender, which must be absolutely free of all other food residues. Just enough distilled water to cover the rotating blades is added, and food and water are blended into a concentrated solution thin enough to be drawn up into the dropper syringe. This solution is poured into a clean cup which is labelled and placed on a tray. Solutions are made from as many of the other foods as can conveniently be tested in one session (it takes about ten minutes to test each food).

Meanwhile, somebody makes a list of each patient's main symptoms and prepares a chart for each similar to the one shown on page 135. The patients should be seated in easy chairs, with an observer sitting beside each one. After the patients have been sitting relaxed for five or ten minutes, their basic resting pulse rate is taken and entered on their charts. In addition, the observer gives the patient a score of o to 3 for each of the symptoms on his or her chart (o = no indication of symptom; 1 = slight indication; 2 = moderate; 3 = severe). Now the tests can begin.

The tray of food extracts, covered with a cloth, is brought in, together with a tray of disposable 10-ml syringes (with the needles removed) that have the millilitres marked off. Paper towels, jugs of distilled water, glasses for each patient to drink from and bowls to be used as spittoons must also be provided. One of the food extracts is drawn into a syringe up to the 1-ml mark. The patient puts his head back and places his tongue against the roof of his mouth. One or two drops from the syringe are put under the patient's tongue. The patient keeps his mouth open for two minutes, then brings his head forward and rinses his mouth out with distilled water. At the end of each test observation and 'turn-off' (see chart), the mouth is rinsed again with water, to leave it clean for the next test.

Now the observer beside each patient takes the pulse again and enters it on the chart after two minutes, watching all the while for signs or reaction. Questioning the patient is not forbidden – in fact it helps – but some of the observations should be purely objective, such as the size of pupils, redness or pallor of skin, signs of restlessness or anxiety, etc.

If the pulse rises or falls 20 beats or more or changes in volume dramatically beneath the testing finger, a reaction must be expected, but some reactions come on without any warning pulse change at all.

In a reaction, symptoms which were minimal or non-existent before the drop went in will appear within a minute or two. The patient may suddenly flush, pupils may dilate or go to pin-points, weeping may start, agitation become apparent and headache or other aches and pains be complained of. Sometimes the patient becomes high in mood, groggy and confused or may fall asleep.

Once the observer is sure that a reaction is well under way, its timing and strength from 1 to 3 is recorded on the chart and then the first 'turn-off' drop can be given, in an attempt to cut the reaction short. Distilled water is drawn up to the 10-ml mark in the syringe, making the solution 1/10th of the original strength, and a drop of that put under

SUBLINGUAL PROVOCATIVE FOOD TESTS

name _Ms A.B._ date _____

ward _____ food _White flour_

0 = none 1 = mild 2 = moderate 3 = severe

signs and symptoms	pre-test	drop goes in	minutes after 2	3	4	turn-offs 1st 1/10	2nd 1/100	3rd 1/1000	oxygen	final
depression	0	1		2	1	1	0	0		
weeping	0	1		2	1	0	0	0		
guilt	0									
anxiety	0									
restless	0	3		3	2	1	0	0		
attempts to run	0									
impatience	0									
hatred, anger	0									
fatigue	0									
sleep	0									
dizzy	0									
confused thinking	0	2		2	1	1	0	0		
wanting to avoid company	0	2		2	2	1	0	0		
inability to concentrate	0	2		2	1	1	0	0		
weakness	0									
hunger	0									
pulse	74	97		104	92	88	80	74		
pupils	●	●		●	●	●	●	●		
skin colour change	0	red		pink	pink	0	0	0		
head down	0	1		1	1	0	0	0		

Example of test score sheet from an actual case

the patient's tongue and left for one to two minutes. This may suffice to turn the reaction off and bring the patient back to normal. If it does not, then the solution is diluted to 1/100th strength by squirting away all but the last 1 ml of the 1/10th solution and drawing up distilled water again to the 10-ml mark. Shake the syringe and use this solution as a further turn-off. Sometimes, in a very severe reaction, it may be necessary to go down to 1/1,000th or even 1/10,000th dilution and then to give inhalations of oxygen or walk the patient up and down in the fresh air before normality (freedom from symptoms) is restored and another test can be begun. With practice, the whole operation can go smoothly and rapidly and the helpers soon get the idea, becoming interested and enthusiastic. With a bit of good humour, a testing session can become like a party game.

Groups I have run on these lines quickly develop a cohesion and life of their own, patients helping each other, offering advice and support, and generally becoming more alive and hopeful.

When all the tests have been done (and of course they have all to be preceded by five days' avoidance of the foods concerned) compatible menus are drawn up for each patient and further testing arranged so as to expand the choice of foods available.

For those people who feel they cannot spare the time either to join a group or to do the open-plate food testing described earlier, modification of Rowe's elimination dieting may be helpful. Try cutting out a whole group of foods commonly found to be allergenic: sugars and cereal grains, for instance. Leave them out for a week or two and see if symptoms abate. In my experience main offenders, besides cereals and sugars, are instant coffee, tea, chocolate, eggs, milk and processed foods. Beer and whisky are often serious offenders for grain-sensitive people. Having avoided these foods, eat them again, one by one, on a test basis, and see if symptoms return. Such a method is not as accurate as the drop-test, but it can and often does bring a reduction in symptoms that is sufficient to make life more bearable again.

Finally, do not forget tobacco. Chronic smokers can test their allergy to tobacco by cutting out smoking for five days, then getting a friend to blow cigarette smoke through a little water in a cup repeatedly, until the solution is brown. One drop of this solution under the tongue will often bring a reaction so devastating that the addict will never wish to smoke again.

chapter nine

When Ivan Illich said in 1974 that the perils inherent in the industrialized production of food now pose perhaps the greatest threat to the health of mankind, he was not exaggerating. Food is man's most intimate contact, far more intimate than copulation. What you eat goes right inside you, is absorbed directly into the bloodstream and carried into every cell in the body, including, most importantly from the point of view of mental health and behaviour, the brain cells.

We are not infinitely adaptable animals, and there is mounting evidence that many of us have already adapted as much as we can to today's increasingly sophisticated and chemically contaminated diet. It is time to call a halt to this appallingly risky experiment in human nutrition and to look again at the relationship between the food we eat and the changing pattern of disease in industrialized countries.

Look how drastically the pattern of disease has changed since the Industrial Revolution began to alter our environment, and particularly our diet. Coronary thrombosis, which now kills about 100,000 people annually in the United Kingdom alone, was unknown to nineteenth-century physicians. Not until 1910 was the first case described in the British medical literature. Now, instead of the devastating epidemics of infectious diseases like typhoid, tuberculosis, cholera and smallpox that used to decimate us before the twentieth century, we have equally devastating epidemics of strokes, high blood pressure, heart attacks, behavioural disorders, allergies and degenerative diseases. All these have taken over now, leaving us little healthier than we were a hundred years ago. What is the reason?

It could be, of course, that we are living longer. But, though there is some validity in that explanation, it is far from the whole story. What we are doing to our food, drink and the air we breathe is the biggest factor of all – I agree with Illich in believing that. Not only is it the least well acknowledged factor, it is also the one we could do most about if we looked at it again in the light of what is now known about allergy to foods and their chemical contaminants.

Earlier I quoted Dr Albert Rowe's 1930 statement that allergy, particularly food allergy, was, after infection, the greatest cause of illness in Westernized society. I now think that allergy has overtaken infection and is the number-one cause.

For the past eighteen years I have been living as far as possible on a Stone-Age-type diet, rich in animal fat and protein and practically free of sugar, cereals and processed carbohydrates: a diet that some of my medical friends assure me should have given me a coronary thrombosis years ago and is bound to kill or cripple me long before I have lived out my normal three score years and ten. On the contrary, at the age of fifty-nine, I am in better health than ever.

The word *allergy*, in the sense in which I have been using it, means an altered reaction, an abnormal reaction, on the part of one or more tissues of the body following exposure to or contact with a nonliving substance, such as a food or chemical. If a person is ill in body, mind, or both and gets well after a five-day fast, then one of the possible causes of his illness is some abnormal reaction to the foods and chemicals he or she has been eating. If the person is then fed on a test basis and it is found that particular foods cause the illness to recur in acute form, it is only logical to suppose that he or she is allergic to those foods. That is the approach I have taken with my patients, stated in the simplest possible terms. The results have astonished even my most sceptical medical colleagues.

As anyone who has actually read Freud's original writings knows, that great man maintained that one day a physiological cause would be found for mental illness. In food and chemical allergy one such demonstrable, physiological cause has at last been found and can be used to good effect by any doctor who takes the trouble to learn about it.

I claim no originality at all in putting forward the details of this approach. All I have done is to read the published works of the many American doctors who have pioneered it (a number of whom I have met). I then tried out their methods, first as a general practitioner and more recently as a psychiatrist, and I have found that they work better than I ever dared to hope. What is so amazing is that everything in this book has been known and written about in medical books and journals since the early 1920s. Yet, up to now, only a handful of doctors in America and Europe have ever bothered to try to investigate and treat patients by this method.

The story of the development of food and chemical allergy as a viable, practical clinical approach in medicine and psychiatry goes back to Americans like Duke, Shannon and Rowe in the early 1920s, who showed that by eliminating certain common items from their patients' diets – wheat, eggs and milk – they were able to clear up long-standing symptoms like headache, asthma and skin eruptions.

Shannon, a paediatrician, published his first cases in 1922 [36]. Rowe began publishing papers about the same time, and his first major book on food allergy was published in 1931 [30].

Hans Selye developed the concept of the general adaptation syndrome to a harmful physical agent, with its three stages: 1 alarm, 2 resistance or adaptation, and 3 exhaustion. Selye's work contributed greatly to the understanding of how patients become ill through failing to adapt to foods and chemicals to which they are allergic. He first published his findings in a 1936 letter to *Nature* [33]. He followed this a few years later with a long, three-part publication in the *American Journal of Allergy* [34].

Herbert Rinkel, who ranks with Rowe and Randolph in the triumvirate of doctors who launched this approach in the United States, discovered the key concept of masked allergy accidentally while trying to cure his own intractable nasal allergy. Masking is the reduction of symptoms by eating a food to which you are allergic within the time (up to three days) that you are still reacting to that particular food. You first feel picked-up and then, later, hung-over. Masking accounts for the addict's craving for his particular food or drink. It clarifies such terms as habituation, inurement, getting used to or tolerance which people use to describe the universal experience of masking in relation to symptoms produced by a food or chemical to which they have unknowingly become allergic or hypersensitive. The mother who tells you that cow's milk made her child vomit soon after it was introduced to the child's diet and boasts that, because she persisted with the milk feeding, her child can now take it and even likes it, is talking about masked food allergy.

In 1971 Randolph's Human Ecology Study Group in Chicago published a pamphlet entitled 'The realities of food addiction'. This is the introductory summary:

Foods . . . eaten daily by the pound and absorbed over a period of two or three days . . . are man's greatest environmental exposures.

Food addiction, which initially is usually confused with normalcy, manifests itself sooner or later in a wide range of physical and/or mental illnesses. This process sets the stage for the development of addictive responses to other more rapidly absorbed and potentially harmful agents.

Food addiction is capable of occurring in anyone. As it usually involves multiple common foods, it is demonstrated most convincingly by preliminary fasting under environmentally controlled conditions, then observing the acute effects resulting from single test re-exposures.

Fasting or avoidance of the addictant for five days or more returns the patient to stage one, the stage of alarm. A single test re-exposure – even, extraordinarily enough, a drop of the food or drink under the tongue – will bring back the chronic symptoms in acute, easily recognizable form. Further weaker drops under the tongue turn the reaction off, probably by a form of quick masking. This method is repeatable and easily taught. Even as I am writing this page, one of the nurses I have trained in the method is carrying out sublingual drop tests on two allergic patients on one of my wards and recording the results, entirely unsupervised by me or any other doctor, in order to help build up compatible diets for the patients to take home.

Once a patient has reached the stage of exhaustion in the battle of adaptation to a particular substance, avoidance is the only remedy known so far. Substances that can aid resistance or block the allergy, when it affects the brain, have yet to be fully evaluated. It is interesting that the most successful major psychiatric tranquillizer, chlorpromazine (Largactil or Thorazine), is chemically derived from an antihistamine, a class of drug used to control the symptoms of hay fever and other allergies. So too was the popular anti-depressant drug imipramine (Tofranil). The pharmaceutical subsidiary of Fisons, the agricultural chemical firm, has already developed a compound, cromoglycate (Intal), which, if taken daily, will prevent or reduce the number of attacks suffered by an asthmatic. I suspect that once the medical profession recognizes the importance of food and chemical allergy in the causation of mental and physical illness, the pharmaceutical industry will step up its efforts to develop drugs that will reverse or block allergic reactions rather than merely reduce the symptoms. The issue of the *Lancet* dated 24 May 1975 carried a favourable report on another anti-allergic agent, Doxantrozole, that has been shown to be effective when taken orally, and Dr Len McEwen of St Mary's Hospital in London has developed a vaccine effective against allergies to many foods.

Dr McEwen is a research pharmacologist working in the Wright-Fleming Institute at St Mary's, the leading allergy unit in Britain. Versed in the bacteriological and immunological approach to allergy pioneered at St Mary's by Sir Alexander Fleming and Sir Almroth Wright, McEwen has incorporated bacteria as well as minute doses of about fifty common foods in his vaccine, which he applies in a plastic cup to a scarified area of the patient's forearm for twenty-four hours three or four times a year. Some of his successes with cases of asthma and hay fever resistant to the conventional pollen-, mould- and dust-based injections, must, I think, be due to his taking bacteria into account in the development of food allergy. I am indebted to him for showing me his methods, which I am beginning to incorporate into my own.

Here are the criteria for spotting food allergy. See how many, if any, of your own symptoms fit in.

1 Illness fluctuates
2 Five symptoms that come and go:
  (a) Swelling of different parts of the body
  (b) Heavy sweating, unrelated to exercise
  (c) Fatigue, not helped by rest
  (d) Bouts of racing pulse
  (e) Marked fluctuations in weight
3 Evidence of food addiction and repetitive menus
4 Other obvious conventional allergies, e.g. hay fever, urticaria, rashes, headache (often morning), asthma
5 Various food-allergic symptoms referred to particular parts of the body:

Head
Nasal catarrh and hay fever
Giddiness
Aphthous ulcers (mouth ulcers)
Halitosis (bad breath)
Headache
Migraine

Chest
Asthmatic wheezing
Tachycardia (racing pulse)

Abdomen
Bloating after food
Irritable colon syndrome
Peptic ulcer syndrome (with no X-ray evidence)

Regional ileitis
Bowel cramps

Genito-urinary
Frequent urination and 'cystitis', without evidence of
 infection
Impotence
Frigidity
Menstrual disorders

Musculo-skeletal
'Fibrositis' (aching muscles)
Arthralgia (aching joints)

Skin
Urticaria (weals or hives)
Itchy rashes that come and go

Mental
Panic attacks and chronic anxiety
Depression
Hypomania (persistent elation unrelated to circumstances)
Hyperkinesis (overactivity)
Purposeless violence
Tension
Thought disorder (delusions and hallucinations)
Alcoholism
Drug addiction

If you have any of these symptoms, your own doctor
should examine you thoroughly, with the help of his
hospital colleagues, to rule out potentially dangerous
causes such as tumours or infections for some of these conditions. *If you have not already done so, please have your doctor
conduct such an examination before applying for tests for food and
chemical allergy.*

Ideally, fasting and testing for food and chemical allergens are not do-it-yourself procedures. With major, disabling symptoms, particularly the psychiatric ones such as acute depression, withdrawal effects during the early days of the fast can be very severe, and the test reactions themselves may require medical attention. Moreover, choosing the foods for testing requires specialized knowledge of sources and methods of processing, which only a doctor interested in this subject will have.

An important point to recognize is that anyone with an allergic background is *potentially* allergic to *anything*, if he or she eats or drinks it often enough. So, if you should work out a menu of 'safe' foods for yourself, try not to repeat any item more than once in three days. Beware if you find you are starting to take a 'safe' food more and more often. You may be becoming allergic to it and therefore eating it addictively. Repetitive eating of a food while still not allergic to it may create an allergy to it. Once the allergy is established, addiction will make you crave it more and more, and leaving it out will give you a hangover for a day or two. Some people, however, can eat the same thing day after day and never become allergic (addicted) to it. When in doubt about a food you thought was safe, cut it out of your diet. Later, after more than five days' avoidance, eat it again on a test basis to see if it makes you unwell.

Finally, if you still find yourself with symptoms after living on your compatible diet, suspect a chemical allergy to something in your home or at work: to the fumes of indoor heaters, gas stoves, traffic exhaust, plastic furniture, synthetic fabrics, or – most common of all – to the pro-pellant in aerosol spray cans. One of my most recent patients was found to be extremely sensitive to all kinds of aerosol sprays – perfumes, deodorants, air fresheners. A few inhalations of any of them caused her to lose control of her muscles and to break out in an itchy rash all over her body. Processed foods, with their high ratio of chemical additives, had the same bad effects, but she had surprisingly few allergies to plain, uncontaminated foods.

It may be necessary to go away to a house in the country where there are no sprays or gas, and to stay there for a week on your compatible diet in order to determine whether allergy to a chemical in the air of your home is the major culprit in your illness.

Sooner or later, government action will *have to* be taken to stop the steadily accelerating drift into a harmful chemical environment. If something effective is not done now to prevent the adaptive breakdown already afflicting more and more people in the West, we shall reach the point of no return, and extinction of our complex, contaminated, improvident society will be inevitable.

References

1 Adolph, E. F., 'General and specific characteristics of physiological adaptations', *American Journal of Physiology, 184,* 1956, pp 18–28

2 Andresen, A. F. R., 'Ulcerative colitis – an allergic phenomenon', *American Journal of Digestive Disease, 9,* 91–8

3 Banting, William, *On Corpulence,* Harrison, London, 1864

4 Brown, E. A. and Colombo, N. J., 'The asthmathogenic effects of odors, smells and fumes', *Annals of Allergy, 12,* 1954, pp 14–24

5 Cannon, Walter B., *The Wisdom of the Body,* Kegan Paul, London, 1932

6 Clark, Harry G. and Randolph, T. G., 'Sodium bicarbonate in the treatment of allergic conditions', *Journal of Laboratory and Clinical Medicine, 44,* 1954, p 914

7 Coca, A. F., *Familial Nonreaginic Food-Allergy,* Charles C. Thomas, Springfield, Illinois and Blackwell Scientific Publications, Oxford, 1942

8 Dicke, W. K., 'Coelike', MD Thesis, University of Utrecht, 1950

9 Dicke, W. K., van de Kamer, J. H. and Weijers, H. A., 'Coeliac disease: presence in wheat of factor having deleterious effect in cases of coeliac disease', *Acta Pediatrica, 42,* January 1953, pp 223–31

10 Dohan, F. C., 'Cereals and schizophrenia', *Acta Psychiatrica Scandinavica, 42,* 1966, pp 125–52; 'Wartime changes in admissions for schizophrenia', *ibid* pp 1–23

11 Dohan, F. C., Grasberger, J. C., Lowell, F. M. *et al.,* 'Relapsed schizophrenics: more rapid improvement on a

milk-and cereal-free diet', *British Journal of Psychiatry*, *115*, May 1969, pp 595–6

12 Donaldson, B., *Strong Medicine*, Cassell, London and Doubleday, New York, 1962

13 Duke, W. W., *Allergy, Asthma, Hay Fever and Allied Manifestations of Reactions*, C. V. Mosby, St Louis, 1925

14 Feingold, Ben, *Why Your Child is Hyperactive*, Random House, New York, 1975

15 Fry, John, *Common Diseases – Their Nature, Incidence and Care*, Medical & Technical Publications Ltd, Lancaster, 1974

16 Haeckel, E., *Generalle Morphologie der Organismen*, G. Reimer, Berlin, 1866

17 Hare, F. W. E., *The Food Factor in Disease*, 2 vols, Longmans, London and New York, 1905

18 *The Genuine Works of Hippocrates*, trans. Francis Adams, Williams and Wilkins Co, Baltimore, 1939

19 Kwok, Robert, 'The Chinese restaurant syndrome', *New England Journal of Medicine*, *278*, 14, 1968, p 796

20 McEwen, L. M., 'Systemic manifestations of hypersensitivity to foods', *Allergologia et Immunopathologia*, Supp. 1, *91*, 1973

21 Mackarness, Richard, 'Stone-Age diet for functional disorders', *Medical World*, *91*, 1959, pp 14–19

22 Mackarness, Richard, *Eat Fat and Grow Slim*, Harvill Press, London, 1958 and Fontana, 1961

23 Piness, G. and Miller, H., 'Allergic manifestations in infancy and childhood', *Archives of Pediatrics*, *42*, 1925, pp 557–62

24 Pirquet, Clemens von, 'Allergie', *Münchener Med. Wochenschrift*, *53*, 1906, p 1457

25 Randolph, T. G., 'Concepts of food allergy important in specific diagnosis', *Journal of Allergy*, *21*, 1950, pp 471–7

26 Randolph, T. G., Rinkel, H. J. and Zeller, M., *Food Allergy*, Charles C. Thomas, Springfield, Illinois, 1951

27 Randolph, T. G., *Human Ecology and Susceptibility to the Chemical Environment*, Charles C. Thomas, Springfield, Illinois, 1962

28 Rinkel, H. J., 'Role of food allergy in internal medicine', *Annals of Allergy*, *2*, 1944, pp 115–24

29 Rinkel, H. J., 'The management of clinical allergy' parts i–iv, *Archives of Otolaryngology*, *76*, *77*, December 1962–March 1963

30 Rowe, A. H., *Food Allergy, Its Manifestations, Diagnosis and Treatment, with a General Discussion of Bronchial Asthma*, Lee & Febiger, Philadelphia, 1931

31 Rowe, A. H., *Clinical Allergy*, Baillière, Tindal & Cox, London, 1937

32 Rowe, A. H., *Elimination Diets and the Patient's Allergies*, Henry Kimpton, London, 1944

33 Selye, H., 'A syndrome produced by diverse nocuous agents', *Nature*, *138*, 1936, p 32

34 Selye, H., 'The general adaptation syndrome and the diseases of adaptation', *American Journal of Allergy*, *17*, 1946

35 Selye, H., *The Stress of Life*, Longmans Green & Co, London, 1957

36 Shannon, W. R., 'Neuropathic manifestations in infants and children as a result of anaphylactic reaction to foods contained in their dietary', *American Journal of Diseases of Children*, *24*, 1922, pp 89–94

37 Truelove, S. C., 'Ulcerative colitis provoked by milk', *British Medical Journal*, *1*, 1961, pp 154–65

Index

Recommended Readings

- Siddhartha by Hermann Hesse, www.bnpublishing.net

- The Anatomy of Success, Nicolas Darvas, www.bnpublishing.net

- The Dale Carnegie Course on Effective Speaking, Personality Development, and the Art of How to Win Friends & Influence People, Dale Carnegie, www.bnpublishing.net

- The Law of Success In Sixteen Lessons by Napoleon Hill (Complete, Unabridged), Napoleon Hill, www.bnpublishing.net

- It Works, R. H. Jarrett, www.bnpublishing.net

- The Art of Public Speaking (Audio CD), Dale Carnegie, wwww.bnpublishing.net

- The Success System That Never Fails (Audio CD), W. Clement Stone, www.bnpublishing.net